Praise for Anthony William

"Anthony doesn't offer gimmicks or fads to finding ultimate health. His recommended foods and cleansing programs are simple and delicious and THEY WORK! If you're done living with pain, fatigue, brain fog, intestinal disorders, and a myriad of other nasty ailments, drop everything and read this (and his other) books. He will quickly bring health and hope back into your life."

— Hilary Swank, Oscar-winning actress

"Celery juice is sweeping the globe. It's impressive how Anthony has created this movement and restored superior health in countless people around the world."

— Sylvester Stallone

"Anthony's understanding of foods, their vibrations, and how they interact with the body never ceases to amaze. Effortlessly he explains the potential harmony or disharmony in our choices in a way anyone can understand. He has a gift. Do your body a favor and treat yourself."

— Pharrell Williams, 13-time Grammy-winning artist and producer

"I've been drinking celery juice every morning for the last six months and feel great! I've noticed a huge difference in my energy levels and digestive system. I even travel now with my juicer so I don't miss out on my daily celery juice!"

— Miranda Kerr, international supermodel, founder and CEO of KORA Organics

"Anthony has turned numerous lives around for the better with the healing powers of celery juice."

— Novak Djokovic, #1-ranked tennis champion in the world

"Anthony is a trusted source for our family. His work in the world is a light that has guided many to safety. He means so much to us."

— Robert De Niro and Grace Hightower De Niro

"While there is most definitely an element of otherworldly mystery to the work he does, much of what Anthony William shines a spotlight on—particularly around autoimmune disease—feels inherently right and true. What's better is that the protocols he recommends are natural, accessible, and easy to do."

— Gwyneth Paltrow, Oscar-winning actress, #1 *New York Times* best-selling author, founder and CEO of GOOP.com

"We are incredibly grateful for Anthony and his passionate dedication to spreading the word about healing through food. Anthony has a truly special gift. His practices have entirely reshaped our perspectives about food and ultimately our lifestyle. Celery juice alone has completely transformed the way we feel and it will always be a part of our morning routine."

— Hunter Mahan, 6-time PGA Tour–winning golfer

"Anthony William is changing and saving the lives of people all over the world with his one-of-a-kind gift. His constant dedication and vast amount of highly advanced information have broken the barriers that block so many in the world from receiving desperately needed truths that science and research have not yet discovered. On a personal level, he has helped both my daughters and me, giving us tools to support our health that actually work. Celery juice is now a part of our regular routine!"

— Lisa Rinna, star of *The Real Housewives of Beverly Hills* and *Days of Our Lives*, *New York Times* best-selling author, designer of the Lisa Rinna Collection

"Anthony is a truly generous person with keen intuition and knowledge about health. I have seen firsthand the transformation he's made in people's quality of life."

— Carla Gugino, star of *Jett*, *The Haunting of Hill House*, *Watchmen*, *Entourage*, *Spy Kids*

"I've been following Anthony for a while now and am always floored (but not surprised) at the success stories from people following his protocols . . . I have been on my own path of healing for many years, jumping from doctor to doctor and specialist to specialist. He's the real deal and I trust him and his vast knowledge of how the thyroid works and the true effects food has on our body. I have directed countless friends, family, and followers to Anthony because I truly believe he possesses knowledge that no doctor out there has. I am a believer and on a true path to healing now and am honored to know him and blessed to know his work. Every endocrinologist needs to read his book on the thyroid!"

— Marcela Valladolid, chef, author, television host

"What if someone could simply touch you and tell you what it is that ails you? Welcome to the healing hands of Anthony William—a modern-day alchemist who very well may hold the key to longevity. His lifesaving advice blew into my world like a healing hurricane, and he has left a path of love and light in his wake. He is hands down the ninth wonder of the world."

— Lisa Gregorisch-Dempsey, *Extra* Senior Executive Producer

"I love Anthony William! My daughters Sophia and Laura gave me his book for my birthday, and I couldn't put it down. The Medical Medium has helped me connect all the dots on my quest to achieve optimal health. Through Anthony's work, I realized the residual Epstein-Barr left over from a childhood illness was sabotaging my health years later. Medical Medium has transformed my life."

— Catherine Bach, *The Young and the Restless*, *The Dukes of Hazzard*

"My recovery from a traumatic spinal crisis several years ago had been steady, but I was still experiencing muscle weakness, a tapped-out nervous system, as well as extra weight. A dear friend called me one evening and strongly recommended I read the book Medical Medium by Anthony William. So much of the information in the book resonated with me that I began incorporating some of the ideas, then I sought and was lucky enough to get a consultation.
The reading was so spot-on, it has taken my healing to an unimagined, deeper, and richer level of health. My weight has dropped healthily, I can enjoy bike riding and yoga, I'm back in the gym, I have steady energy, and I sleep deeply. Every morning when following my protocols, I smile and say, 'Whoa, Anthony William! I thank you for your restorative gift . . . Yes!'"

— Robert Wisdom, *Ballers*, *The Alienist*, *Rosewood*, *Nashville*, *The Wire*, *Ray*

"In this world of confusion, with constant noise in the health and wellness field, I rely on Anthony's profound authenticity. His miraculous, true gift rises above it all to a place of clarity."

— Patti Stanger, host of *Million Dollar Matchmaker*

"I rely on Anthony William for my and my family's health. Even when doctors are stumped, Anthony always knows what the problem is and the pathway for healing."

— Chelsea Field, *NCIS: New Orleans*, *Secrets and Lies*, *Without a Trace*, *The Last Boy Scout*

"Anthony William brings a dimension to medicine that deeply expands our understanding of the body and of ourselves. His work is part of a new frontier in healing, delivered with compassion and with love."

— Marianne Williamson, #1 *New York Times* best-selling author of *Healing the Soul of America*, *The Age of Miracles*, and *A Return to Love*

"Anthony William is a generous and compassionate guide. He has devoted his life to supporting people on their healing path."

— Gabrielle Bernstein, #1 *New York Times* best-selling author of *The Universe Has Your Back*, *Judgment Detox*, and *Miracles Now*

"Information that WORKS. That's what I think of when I think of Anthony William and his pro-found contributions to the world. Nothing made this fact so clear to me as seeing him work with an old friend who had been struggling for years with illness, brain fog, and fatigue. She had been to countless doctors and healers and had gone through multiple protocols. Nothing worked. Until Anthony talked to her, that is . . . from there, the results were astounding. I highly recommend his books, lectures, and consultations. Don't miss this healing opportunity!"

— Nick Ortner, *New York Times* best-selling author of *The Tapping Solution for Manifesting Your Greatest Self* and *The Tapping Solution*

"Esoteric talent is only a complete gift when it's shared with moral integrity and love. Anthony William is a divine combination of healing, giftedness, and ethics. He's a real-deal healer who does his homework and shares it in true service to the world."

— Danielle LaPorte, best-selling author of *White Hot Truth* and *The Desire Map*

"Anthony is a seer and a wellness sage. His gift is remarkable. With his guidance I've been able to pinpoint and address a health issue that's been plaguing me for years."

— Kris Carr, *New York Times* best-selling author of *Crazy Sexy Juice*, *Crazy Sexy Kitchen*, and *Crazy Sexy Diet*

"Twelve hours after receiving a heaping dose of self-confidence masterfully administered by Anthony, the persistent ringing in my ears of the last year . . . began to falter. I am astounded, grateful, and happy for the insights offered on moving forward."

— Mike Dooley, *New York Times* best-selling author of *Infinite Possibilities* and scribe of *Notes from the Universe*

"Whenever Anthony William recommends a natural way of improving your health, it works. I've seen this with my daughter, and the improvement was impressive. His approach of using natural ingredients is a more effective way of healing."

— Martin D. Shafiroff, financial advisor, past recipient of #1 Broker in America ranking by WealthManagement.com and #1 Wealth Advisor ranking by Barron's

"Anthony William's invaluable advice on preventing and combating disease is years ahead of what's available anywhere else."

— Richard Sollazzo, M.D., New York board-certified oncologist, hematologist, nutritionist, and anti-aging expert and author of *Balance Your Health*

MEDICAL MEDIUM

THYROID HEALING

ALSO BY ANTHONY WILLIAM

Medical Medium: Secrets Behind Chronic and Mystery Illness and How to Finally Heal

*Medical Medium Life-Changing Foods: Save Yourself and the Ones You Love
with the Hidden Healing Powers of Fruits & Vegetables*

*Medical Medium Liver Rescue: Answers to Eczema, Psoriasis, Diabetes,
Strep, Acne, Gout, Bloating, Gallstones, Adrenal Stress, Fatigue, Fatty Liver,
Weight Issues, SIBO & Autoimmune Disease*

*Medical Medium Celery Juice: The Most Powerful Medicine
of Our Time Healing Millions Worldwide*

*Medical Medium Cleanse To Heal: Healing Plans for Sufferers of Anxiety, Depression,
Acne, Eczema, Lyme, Gut Problems, Brain Fog, Weight Issues, Migraines, Bloating, Vertigo,
Psoriasis, Cysts, Fatigue, PCOS, Fibroids, UTI, Endometriosis & Autoimmune*

The above are available at your local bookstore, or may be ordered by visiting:

Hay House USA: www.hayhouse.com®
Hay House Australia: www.hayhouse.com.au
Hay House UK: www.hayhouse.co.uk
Hay House India: www.hayhouse.co.in

MEDICAL MEDIUM

THYROID HEALING

THE TRUTH BEHIND HASHIMOTO'S, GRAVES', INSOMNIA, HYPOTHYROIDISM, THYROID NODULES & EPSTEIN-BARR

ANTHONY WILLIAM

HAY HOUSE, INC.
Carlsbad, California • New York City
London • Sydney • New Delhi

Published in the United States by: Hay House, Inc.: www.hayhouse.com®
Published in Australia by: Hay House Australia Pty. Ltd.: www.hayhouse.com.au
Published in the United Kingdom by: Hay House UK, Ltd.: www.hayhouse.co.uk
Published in India by: Hay House Publishers India: www.hayhouse.co.in

Cover design: Vibodha Clark
Interior design: Bryn Starr Best
Interior illustration design: Vibodha Clark
Recipe photos: Ashleigh & Britton Foster
Indexer: Jay Kreider

Library of Congress has cataloged the earlier edition as follows:

Names: William, Anthony, author.
Title: Medical medium thyroid healing : the truth behind Hashimoto's,
   Graves', insomnia, hypothyroidism, thyroid nodules & Epstein-Barr /
   Anthony William.
Description: Carlsbad, California : Hay House, Inc., 2017.
Identifiers: LCCN 2017029720 | ISBN 9781401948368 (hardback)
Subjects: LCSH: Thyroid gland--Diseases. | Thyroid
   gland--Diseases--Alternative treatment. | Self-care, Health--Popular
   works. | BISAC: HEALTH & FITNESS / Alternative Therapies. | HEALTH &
   FITNESS / Healthy Living. | MEDICAL / Endocrinology & Metabolism.
Classification: LCC RC655 .W485 2017 | DDC 616.4/4--dc23 LC record available at https://lccn.loc.gov/2017029720

Tradepaper ISBN: 978-1-4019-4837-5
E-book ISBN: 978-1-4019-4838-2
Audiobook ISBN: 978-1-4019-5517-5

11 10 9 8 7 6 5 4 3 2
1st edition, November 2017
2nd edition, June 2021

Printed in China

For all those who have struggled, suffered, and been let down, forgotten, pushed aside, ignored, or betrayed. For those who have fought and battled, persevered, healed, or not healed yet. I stand alongside you. We can rise above it all together with knowledge, wisdom, truth, love, and, most importantly, compassion.

CONTENTS

FOREWORD

What will you find in this jewel of a book? A fascinating and innovative approach to thyroid disease. Thanks to Anthony William and the voice speaking directly to him, you will be given an outpouring of new information about thyroid disease, as well as safe and effective ways to recover.

As a USC-trained gynecologist and pioneer in the field of bioidentical hormones for women, I am always seeking the root "core causes" of illness and decline. I have treated thousands of patients for thyroid disease, and I believe that only half the people who suffer from it in the United States are ever accurately diagnosed. In my professional opinion, it's possible that 7 out of 10 people in this country suffer from thyroid disease. By reading this significant book, you will have much more insight as to your own diagnosis and have the resources needed to stop this problem in its tracks. Since reading Anthony's *Medical Medium Thyroid Healing*, I certainly have new insights and solutions to bring to my tough cases. Indeed, Anthony is exactly right when he writes that not all patients respond to thyroid hormones the way we might expect or hope.

As a medical doctor, if I had a wise and accurate voice speaking to me about my patients' illnesses like Anthony William does, I would consider it a pure miracle. Many of my colleagues would be grateful for this inside help, too, although I don't think the medical profession as a whole would consider this quite so favorably. I can't quite understand why! One of the leading causes of death in the United States comes from prescribed medications and current medical treatments. We blast patients with antibiotics, and look at the thousands of deaths due to antibiotic resistance per year that result. We plummet our cancer patients' immunity with drugs that cause more cancer later. Every day I see the harmful effects of the birth control pill on young women's hormones. *Agh!* I am as frustrated as you are.

To make matters worse, do you know that medical treatments lag 25 years behind scientific medical knowledge? In the information technology (IT) field, this means people today would still be told to buy clunky, quarter-century-old Apple II's, in spite of sophisticated computers being available. Who would consider that a smart purchase? One of my friends was an esteemed CEO in a top high-tech company, managing thousands of people and factories across the globe. At the height of his career, he developed an aggressive brain tumor. In spite of receiving care from top medical facilities in the United States, he was shocked by the lack of innovative approaches. While the IT industry had solved incredibly complex and seemingly impossible problems, treatment for his type of cancer hadn't really advanced for more than a decade. He was a wonderful, kind man, and lamented with real frustration that if he ran his company the way doctors practiced medicine, his company would be bankrupt in less than a month. When I see patients misdiagnosed and mismanaged by traditional "old-style" medicine, I feel the same disbelief.

And that is why I have read with fascination and an open mind Anthony's *Medical Medium* and this new book, *Medical Medium Thyroid Healing*. Patients need answers now and can't wait for answers that might come in two decades. Besides, I know with certainty that answers don't just come out of the lab or from clinical trials. Call it *Consciousness*, *God*, *the Voice*, *the Field*, or whatever you wish; Anthony is tapped into a source of knowledge, wisdom, and healing of enormous value.

Researchers, medical doctors, and other scientists are extremely interested in the connection between viruses and disease processes. For years, I have been reading about how viruses are implicated in unexpected diseases and future cancers. For example,

in the early 1960s, EBV was identified as the probable cause of a rare lymphoma, and now medical evidence shows that the virus is linked to Hodgkin's disease, autoimmune diseases, MS, and hundreds of thousands of cases of cancer per year. Still, we know very little about *how* viruses are involved with these issues and how to effectively treat conditions that arise from viruses.

In this book, Anthony brings innovative concepts to thyroid disease—revealing EBV as the significant core cause. He explodes many of the thyroid myths you may have heard and offers brilliant, in fact enlightened, answers. The supplements, dietary wisdom, herbs, and thyroid healing techniques are all unique and hold tremendous value. He tells us we don't have to suffer from thyroid disease, and I wholeheartedly agree with him. Since reading *Medical Medium Thyroid Healing*, I have expanded my approach and treatments of thyroid disease and am seeing enormous value for patients. The results are rewarding and gratifying.

Thank you, dear Anthony, for using your extraordinary and blessed gifts to help those who suffer. I am grateful for your courage, dedication, and generosity of service to humanity. May the multitudes, including the entire medical community, hear your voice and the voice that guides you!

Prudence Hall, M.D.
Founder and medical director, The Hall Center

A NOTE FOR YOU

Chronic illness is at an all-time high. In America alone, more than 250 million people are sick or dealing with mystery symptoms. These are people leading diminished lives with no explanation—or explanations that don't sit right or that make them feel even worse. You may be one of them. If so, you can attest that medical science is still puzzling through what's behind the epidemic of mystery symptoms and suffering.

Let me be clear that I revere good medical science. There are incredibly gifted and talented doctors, surgeons, nurses, technicians, researchers, chemists, and more doing profound work in both conventional and alternative medicine. I've had the privilege of working with some of them. Thank God for these compassionate healers. Learning how to understand our world through rigorous, systematic inquiry is one of the highest pursuits imaginable.

Like any human pursuit, medical science is still a work in progress. It's constantly evolving, and so theories that one day seem like the be-all and end-all can be revealed the next day to be obsolete. What this translates to is: science doesn't have every answer yet.

We've already waited 100-plus years for real insights from medical communities into thyroid problems, and they haven't come. You shouldn't have to wait another 10, 20, 30, or more years for scientific research to find the real answers. If you're stuck in bed, dragging through your days, or feeling lost about your health, you shouldn't have to go through one more day of it, let alone another decade. You shouldn't have to watch your children go through it, either—and yet millions do.

That's why Spirit of the Most High, God's expression of compassion, came into my life when I was four years old: to teach me how to see the true causes of people's suffering and to get that information out into the world. If you'd like to know more about my origins, you'll find my story in *Medical Medium: Secrets Behind Chronic and Mystery Illness and How to Finally Heal*. The short version is that Spirit constantly speaks into my ear with clarity and precision, as if a friend were standing beside me, filling me in on the symptoms of everyone around me. Plus, Spirit taught me from an early age to see physical scans of people, like supercharged MRI scans that reveal all blockages, illnesses, infections, trouble areas, and past problems.

We see you. We know what you're up against. And we don't want you to go through it a moment longer. My life's work is to deliver this information to you, so that you can be elevated above the sea of confusion—the noise and rhetoric of today's health fads and trends—in order to regain your health and navigate life on your own terms.

The material in this book is authentic, the real deal, all for your benefit. This book is not like other health books. There's so much packed in here, you may want to come back and read it again to make sure you get all the information. Sometimes this information will seem the opposite of what you've heard before, and sometimes it will be close to other sources, with subtle and critical differences. The common thread is that it's the truth. It's not repackaged or recycled theory made to sound like a new understanding of thyroid health. The information here doesn't come from interest groups, medical funding with strings attached, botched research, lobbyists, internal kickbacks, persuaded belief systems, private panels of influencers, health field payoffs, or trendy traps.

The above hurdles get in the way of medical research and science making the leaps and bounds it's meant to in understanding chronic illness. When outside sources have a vested interest in obscuring certain truths, then precious research time and money get spent in unproductive areas. Certain discoveries that would truly advance the treatment of chronic illness get ignored and lose funding. The scientific data we think of as absolute can, instead, be skewed—contaminated and manipulated, then treated by other thyroid experts as law, even though it's inherently flawed.

To go with the facts and figures about thyroid illness in the pages to come, you won't find citations or mentions of scientific studies that have spawned from unproductive sources. You don't need to worry that this information will be proven wrong or superseded, as you do with other health books, because all of the health information I share here comes from a pure, untampered with, advanced, clean source—a higher source: the Spirit of Compassion. There's nothing more healing than compassion.

If you're someone who only believes in what science has to say, know that I like science, too. Also know that science and the thyroid remain very distant from each other in this day and age. The thyroid is still a medical mystery. The scientific studies about this gland are vague, and they lack conclusive answers about the cause of thyroid illness. Unlike many other areas of science, which are strongly founded in weights and measures, scientific thinking about the thyroid is still all theoretical—and today's theories hold very little truth, which is why so many people are still dealing with thyroid illness. Scientific understanding and the thyroid don't have a lot in common yet; they're distinctly divided.

Once upon a time, we lived by the rule of authority. We were told that the earth was flat, and then that the sun revolved around the earth, so we believed it. Those theories weren't fact, and yet people treated them like they were. People living back then didn't feel like life was backwards; it was just the way life was. Anyone who spoke out against the status quo seemed like a fool. Then came the paradigm shift of science. The questioners—the committed researchers and thinkers—the ones who all along hadn't been content to take a "fact" at face value finally proved that analysis could open the door to a much deeper, truer understanding of our world.

Now, science has become the new authority. In some cases, this saves lives. Surgeons now use sterile tools, for example, because they understand the risk of contamination that surgeons of old didn't realize. Just because of certain advancements, though, we can't stop questioning. It's time for another paradigm shift. "Because science" isn't enough of an answer when it comes to chronic illness. Is it *good* science? What was the funding behind it? Was the sample size diverse enough? Big enough? Were the controls handled ethically? Were enough factors considered? Were the measurement tools advanced enough? Does the analysis stamped on the results tell a different story than the numbers themselves? Was there bias? Did an influencer put a thumb on the scale?

Let's be honest. Even today's science in those areas we think to be concrete sometimes shows cracks. If you've heard about recalls of hip replacement parts or hernia mesh, you know what I'm talking about. These are tangible items that were designed with exacting scientific standards, then went through rigorous scientific testing before being put to use, and even that highly scientific process wasn't guaranteed. Certain products developed unforeseen problems, and an area of science that seemed indisputable turned out to be fallible. Think, then, what kind of uncertainty remains in scientific understanding of the thyroid and its true functions. This isn't a device that can be held in your hand, measured, and analyzed. It's an active part of the human body, and we all know the human body to be one of the greatest miracles and mysteries of life. Again, science is a human pursuit and a work in progress, especially when that work involves decoding the human body. It takes constant vigilance, receptiveness, and adaptability to keep that work truly progressing.

If you've never struggled with your health, suffering for years with no answers for your condition, or if you feel cemented within a certain medical, scientific, or nutritional belief system with relation to the thyroid, I hope that you'll approach the chapters to come with curiosity and an open heart. The meaning behind today's widespread thyroid illness is so much bigger than anyone has yet discovered. What you're about to read is unlike any information about the thyroid you've seen before. This information has helped tens of thousands of people over the past decades.

Since I first started to share Spirit's information, I've been so blessed to see it make a difference for these people. With the publication of the Medical Medium book series, I've been beyond moved to see this information reach the wider world and help thousands more.

I've also noticed that some of these messages have been manipulated as certain career-driven individuals try to climb the ladder of acclaim and notoriety. This approach gets at people's core, raw nerve of suffering and takes advantage of it.

This is not how the gift I was given was ever meant to be used. We love it when people become experts on the health information I share and when they spread the compassionate message far and wide in the name of truly helping others. I am so thankful for this. What gets dangerous is when that information is tampered with—intermixed and twisted with trendy misinformation, changed just enough so that it sounds original, or blatantly poached and attributed to seemingly credible sources that are anemic of the truth. I say this because I want you to know to protect yourself and your loved ones from the misguidance out there.

This book is not repetition of everything you've already read. It's not about realizing the thyroid is behind all your health problems, nor is it about putting a spin on a trendy high-protein diet to keep symptoms at bay. This information is fresh—an entirely new perspective on the symptoms holding back so many people in life, and an entirely new perspective on how to heal.

I get it if you're wary. We react, we judge, that's what we do. It can be an instinct that protects us in certain circumstances; sometimes, it gets us through life. In this case, I hope you'll reconsider. You may judge yourself out of learning the truth. You could lose the opportunity to help yourself or somebody else.

So fasten your seat belts with me here. We are all in this together with getting people better, and I want you to become the new expert in thyroid health. Thank you for coming with me on this healing journey and taking the time to read this book. Learning the truth will change everything for you and the ones around you.

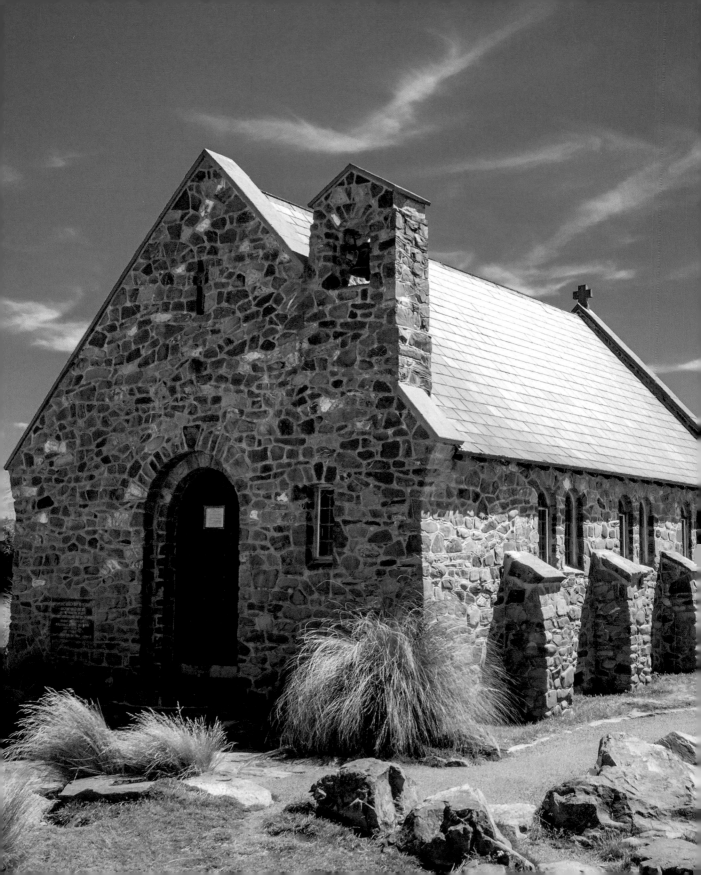

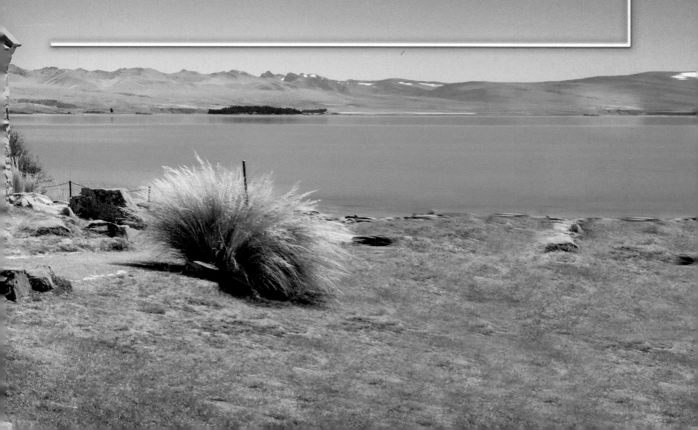

PART I

THYROID
REVELATIONS

CHAPTER 1

The Truth about Your Thyroid

You wake early on the big day. You dress with care, eat as much breakfast as you can stomach, leave a message for your boss to remind her you'll be in late. In the car on the way to your doctor's office, you feel a flicker of hope at the thought that the next time you're behind the wheel, you'll have a little more control over your life.

You may finally have an answer about why you're losing sleep, unable to manage your weight, battling brain fog, watching your hair thin, or dealing with constant fatigue. *At last,* you think, *some insight into the hot flashes, cold hands and feet, brittle nails, dry skin, heart flutters, restless legs, impaired memory, eye floaters, muscle weakness, hormonal fluctuations, dizziness, tingles and numbness, ringing or buzzing in the ears, aches and pains, anxiety, depression.* In the waiting room, you can barely concentrate on the magazine in your lap as you listen for your name to be called.

The moment arrives. You're led to the exam room, where you take a seat and try to breathe slowly. Several minutes later, the doctor walks in, and after a moment of friendly small talk, issues the verdict: "You have Hashimoto's thyroiditis."

There's an element of relief in having a name for what ails you . . . and yet that name doesn't offer much of a clue about what the problem is. "What is that?" you ask.

"The blood work we just got back showed the heightened presence of thyroid antibodies. Along with your elevated levels of thyroid-stimulating hormone, or TSH, your enlarged thyroid gland that showed up in your last exam, and the hypothyroid symptoms you've exhibited, everything indicates that your immune system has become confused. This is called an autoimmune response; it means your body is attacking your thyroid as though it were a foreign presence. It's inflaming the gland and destroying it over time, reducing your thyroid function bit by bit."

Relief fades as you picture this small, innocent gland in your neck under attack from your own immune system. You almost wish this diagnosis were like a pair of shoes you ordered online that you could return once you realized they pinched your toes. *These didn't fit,* you'd indicate on the return label, and then you'd be free of them, free to find a shoe that felt right. Instead, you try to face reality. "How did this happen?"

"It could be that you have a genetic susceptibility to autoimmunity, triggered off by environmental factors such as bacteria, diet, or stress."

"Why would the body ever attack itself, though? Why would it get confused?"

"Well," your doctor says, "the exact cause of autoimmune disease is still unknown." He offers a sympathetic smile. "But research is making strides every day. Now let's talk about medication."

As you drive away from the doctor's office, it's not control you feel; it's betrayal. How could your own body have let you down like this? What did you do wrong to deserve an immune system that's gone haywire? You don't know what you can trust anymore if you can't trust your body to be on your side.

Maybe the scenario above doesn't quite describe your thyroid story. Perhaps instead you've been given a diagnosis of Graves' disease—an autoimmune disease, your doctor says, that throws your thyroid into overdrive.

Or you've been told you have primary hypothyroidism, the underproduction of thyroid hormones, either indicated by a blood test or intuited by a functional medicine doctor who can read the signs. Perhaps you've been told you have a thyroid nodule, a cyst, or even a tumor. Asked why any of this has happened, your doctor answers that you may be aging prematurely—a sobering message, especially if you're only in your 20s or 30s.

Maybe the doctor doesn't stop at a thyroid diagnosis. On top of Hashimoto's or Graves' or hypothyroidism or hyperthyroidism or thyroiditis or growths, you hear that you have Lyme disease, rheumatoid arthritis (RA), or fibromyalgia, or that you're going through perimenopause or menopause. Others may jokingly call you a "basket case," or a hypochondriac, which hurts more than they know given that you'd like nothing better than to be problem-free. It can feel like you're never truly heard.

Perhaps when you first visited the doctor, nothing showed up as wrong in your tests or physical exam. You then visited practitioner after practitioner as you looked for answers, and in the end, you still couldn't find them. You started to lose trust in your doctors *and* yourself. Convinced for a time that your symptoms were all in your head, you've since educated yourself with all the latest literature and come to your own conclusions about what's going on with your health. You've tried a change in diet and felt some relief, though each day is still a bit of a struggle; you still don't quite feel like yourself.

Or it could be that you've been too nervous to visit the doctor about your fatigue, anxiety, brain fog, and dizziness. You've read a couple of articles about the thyroid and wondered if that could be what ails you.

Alternatively, you could be the loved one of someone with persistent, unexplainable symptoms or an identified thyroid ailment. You witness from the sidelines how miserable-making this chronic illness is and wish you could make it all go away and bring back the healthy, vital friend or family member you used to know.

Or it may be that you're the doctor whose heart breaks to see patient after patient in chronic pain or discomfort. You stay on top of the new theories of autoimmunity and thyroid health. You read between the lines with symptoms, don't take blood work as a final answer, offer your patients the latest tools to manage chronic illness, and observe when medication doesn't offer relief, all the time waiting for that breakthrough study that will once and for all solve the mysteries of the thyroid.

If your experience has been similar to any of the above scenarios, you're not alone—you are one among millions confronting the mysterious symptoms that medical communities have begun to connect with thyroid illness. While your story is your own, and the particulars of what you've been through are unique and personal, you stand united with a brave and tireless troop that will not settle for anything less than the greater truth about thyroid health.

Despite the difficulties of your individual experience, you are driven forward. No matter how many times you hear that autoimmune disease is the body attacking itself, no matter how many authorities say that thyroid problems are genetic, no matter how often others have doubted your suffering, or you've doubted yourself and worried that you're defective, or wondered if you're just not trying hard enough at life, you are propelled by a nagging sense that something here can't be quite right.

Why would your body attack itself? If thyroid problems are genetic, why have they only become widespread in recent generations? How could it be possible that all of your physical suffering is in your head, or some sort of cosmic payback?

There must be a bigger explanation, you reason. There must be revelations that will make it all make sense—you know it in your heart.

And you're right.

THE BLAME GAME

Rest assured, your symptoms and illness are not your fault.

Got that? I'll say it again, because the conditioning is so strong in the opposite direction: *your symptoms and illness are not your fault.*

You did not create your illness. You did not attract or manifest it. You did not imagine it. You're not sick because you're crazy, lazy, weak-willed, defective, or bored. You did not bring your symptoms upon yourself by thinking the wrong thoughts or fixating too much on fear. You don't come from a faulty family line. You are not subconsciously holding yourself back from healing because you secretly crave the attention of being

sick. Your suffering is not a punishment from God or the universe, or karma coming back to get you for something you did in this or any other lifetime.

Similarly, your body has not let you down. Thyroid symptoms and illnesses are not your body rebelling against you. It would never betray you. All your body does is work night and day to support you—because *your body loves you unconditionally.*

The most advanced thyroid information out there still misses these key truths. Why? Because we live in a society of blame. As humans, we try to fill in blanks whether we have the right solution or not. Mysteries of the universe are one thing— if we don't have answers about time or space, we can usually live with that as we wait for them to become clear over generations. When it's an unknown that affects our daily lives, on the other hand—say, in the form of aches and pains—then an absence of answers tends to distress us.

So we fill in the blank; when anything goes wrong, we want an explanation as soon as possible. If an assignment at work gets completed incorrectly, for example, everyone wants to know right away whose fault it was. This is based on noble principles: responsibility and accountability. The faster we have answers, we reason, the better we can insure ourselves against a similar mess-up in the future.

What if we end up blaming the wrong source, though? What if, in the rush to figure out why the data on the spreadsheet is skewed, a manager speculates that it was you, the CEO, who gave bad instructions in the first place? What if, for years going forward, everyone mistrusts you when you give out assignments, and you even mistrust yourself? It may make everyone feel more comfortable, in an odd way, to have an answer to point to about why an assignment went awry.

Only—what if it's not the right answer? What if the whole time everyone was pointing at you, the truth was that you'd given flawless instructions, and your staff should have taken the time to determine that a computer bug was the real problem?

That is the world of thyroid illness right now. The idea of not having an explanation for why an overwhelming segment of the population is in long-term pain or discomfort goes against the authoritative image that the medical establishment feels duty-bound to uphold. And so, in the absence of answers, research develops theories such as autoimmunity that place the blame on your body. These medical misconceptions are the *Great Mistakes* of chronic illness, and we'll explore them in detail in Part II of this book. They're well-intentioned: medical science wants to hand you a reason why you're dealing with insomnia, uncontrollable weight gain, or overwhelming fatigue—so you don't have to live in mystery.

Trouble is, these theories often hatch and catch on quickly, then once a theory has been repeated too often and stuck around for too long, it gets mistaken for fact. So medical research operates on the assumption that the theory of autoimmunity is correct, and goes forward exploring the various reasons why the immune system would attack the thyroid. This won't lead to answers, because autoimmune disease is not the body attacking itself—nor is thyroid disease a simple matter of aging, genetics, thinking the wrong thoughts, fixating on certain emotions, or eating foods that trigger inflammation.

Getting a thyroid diagnosis is difficult at any age. Getting a heap of diagnoses and feeling like you're somehow malfunctioning at your core is a burden. So is dealing with mystery symptoms without receiving any sort of name for what's happening to your mind and body.

When you're in your later years, it can feel like an unfair hurdle. Just when some of your obligations are tapering off and you're supposed to get a chance to enjoy life, here come these symptoms to get in your way.

When you're in your 30s, 40s, or 50s, a thyroid problem can feel like you're getting old before your time. The life you've worked so hard to build—the family you've made for yourself, the career—suddenly feels like it could fall apart. You worry about how you can care for everyone you're supposed to care for and stay on top of all you're supposed to do.

And when you're just becoming an adult, the onset of symptoms can feel like a life sentence. At the beginning of a marriage or career, or before you've even had time to start a family or embark on your professional life, you're suddenly sidelined, wondering how in the world you'll be able to support yourself or start and maintain relationships.

At any stage of life, you are already dealing with so much. The last thing you need is to feel like your illness is your own doing—especially because that's far from the truth. So let's take self-blame out of the equation right now. Let's add up the real factors behind thyroid illness so you can finally discover the solution to heal.

THE VIRAL THYROID

Hopefully in two or three decades, medical communities will have the tests and the answers to offer you true relief. If you're suffering right now, though, I doubt you feel you have 20 or 30 years to wait. You've already waited long enough. You've struggled long enough. You've been patient long enough. The time has finally come to arm yourself with the truth, to learn the answers about what's been holding you back.

If you've been diagnosed with Hashimoto's, hypothyroidism, or any other thyroid issue, chances are extremely high that you're not getting the most effective treatment—because without true insight into what causes thyroid illness, medical communities aren't yet able to offer remedies that heal the underlying problem.

And if you've been tested for thyroid issues and the results have come back normal, you could still be suffering with an under- or overactive thyroid gland and not know it—because thyroid testing is not yet entirely accurate.

Some enlightened practitioners are beginning to catch on to this second point. They've seen so many patients present with classic hypothyroid symptoms, despite tests that come back with no indication that anything's wrong, that they've come to the correct conclusion that many more people are suffering with thyroid problems than traditional diagnostics would lead us to believe. To this advanced medical crowd, thyroid illness has begun to reveal itself as an epidemic.

Unfortunately, even the most advanced thyroid information out there today is not enough. Not only is it not enough; much of it is wrong. Because thyroid disease is still misunderstood, even the latest books on thyroid health are outdated before they hit the shelves. The experts consulted on today's up-to-the-minute news programs still share thyroid theories that should be considered behind the times.

I wish the answers were already out there to get you better! And yet they're not—you need to know this so you don't have to waste your precious time combing through the resources out there, which are based on theories of chronic illness that should be deemed antiquated by now. If a book tells you that Hashimoto's and Graves' happen because the body is attacking itself—which is what the latest releases say—it's best to think of it as an antique. Trying to make sense of

thyroid theories might as well be called antique shopping. These theories are cute collectibles, maybe, a glimpse into old-fashioned modes of thought. They aren't going to help you in the present moment.

Though the information you'll find elsewhere is meant to help, it's leading people down a wayward path. Why wayward, if these sources are finally zeroing in on the thyroid? Two reasons: (1) these sources still operate on the premise that autoimmune disease is the body attacking itself—which is far from the truth, as we'll explore in detail soon, and (2) the more focus the thyroid itself gets, the less inclined people are to step back and think about the bigger picture.

And there's a much bigger picture.

Today's theories have only been looking at the decoy, like a hunter's wooden duck placed in a pond to gather a flock so they'll make for easy targets. This decoy—the false concept that the thyroid is to blame for countless ills—is a distraction. If we take away the binoculars and move to higher ground, we'll see that there's a safe haven for the birds that know to look for it, just like you can save yourself and the ones you love by seeking out the spot where the real thyroid truth resides.

Are people's thyroids under attack? Yes. Is the thyroid an important aspect of health? More than anyone knows. Are compromised thyroids the reason millions of people are sick? No.

Here's the pivotal truth that goes by unnoticed in medical journals, on the Internet, and in the latest literature: A thyroid problem is not the ultimate reason for a person's illness. **A problematic thyroid is *yet one more symptom.***

Thyroid ailments are so much bigger than this one small gland in the neck. Thyroid problems don't explain the myriad issues a person may experience; the thyroid is not the ultimate connection that makes it all make sense. It's something much more pervasive in the body, something *in*vasive, that's responsible for the laundry list of symptoms attributed to thyroid disease: the *thyroid virus*.

Everybody who has this common virus is either already experiencing thyroid problems or on their way. And the virus doesn't just go after the thyroid gland. By the time it's gotten to your thyroid, the virus has already reached its third stage—and been troublesome for your health in its earlier stages, whether you've felt its effects or not. The virus causes many symptoms and conditions beyond what's associated with the thyroid, and so, in fact, all of your health problems may point back to this single source. Now that it's in the thyroid, the virus doesn't stop. Its goal is to go even further and compromise your nervous system, causing dozens of mystery symptoms and wreaking further havoc on your health.

Except now that you have access to the greater truth in this book, you have the power to stop it.

In the coming chapters of Part I, "Thyroid Revelations," we'll go into detail about the thyroid virus—how it works, how it causes your symptoms, and what you need to know if you've had thyroid testing or tried medication for it. In Part II, "The Great Mistakes in Your Way," we examine the major misconceptions that shape today's misunderstanding of chronic symptoms and illness—and get in the way of healing. In Part III, "Thyroid Resurrection," you'll discover a tool kit for healing. We'll look at what to know if you've had all or part of your thyroid removed, how to halt the virus in its tracks, and secrets to bringing your thyroid—and the rest of your body—back to health and vitality. This includes the very special 90-Day Thyroid Rehab, along with recipes geared toward thyroid healing.

Finally, in Part IV, "Secrets of Sleep," we'll help you get to the bottom of your sleep issues, from waking in the night to not feeling rested when you get up in the morning to not being able to fall asleep in the first place. Troubled sleep is often cited as a symptom of thyroid problems, when the truth is that insomnia goes far beyond a compromised thyroid. Sleep is still a mystery to medical communities, and it's such a critical component of healing from the thyroid virus and safeguarding your health for the future, so it gets its own in-depth section. We all deserve plenty of restful sleep, and it's available to us if we know how to crack the code.

THE NEW THYROID EXPERT: YOU

In this book are the definitive answers you've been waiting for all along. They are the answers from a higher source about what's led you to this place in your life and how you can turn it all around. Already, you have set yourself on the path to healing. Learning the truth is the first great step.

By the time you've reached the last page, you will have expert knowledge about the thyroid—knowledge that supersedes the theories out there. You will be more informed than anyone on the thyroid circuit. After all, what is a thyroid expert? Is it someone who's well-versed on what's been hypothesized? Or is it someone who understands the full scope of what *is*? Soon, you'll understand the reality of what's going on with your thyroid—and the rest of your body—and you'll be able to use that truth to help yourself heal. *You* will be the thyroid expert.

It doesn't end there. As you transform, others will bear witness; they will ask for your secrets. At the grocery store, at the bookstore, online, or among friends and family, you'll be able to lead others to the thyroid truth. You will contribute to a true healing movement. Your expertise will help so many, more than you'll ever even know.

Now let's begin.

CHAPTER 2

Thyroid Virus Triggers

If you're dealing with a thyroid issue, you've probably asked yourself certain questions: *How did this happen? Why me? Why now?*

And I'm sure that already, before your symptoms, you were no stranger to hardship in one way or another. We go through so much in life. Breakups, betrayals, the passing of loved ones, caring for sick family members, financial strain, injuries, and more—since I was young, I've been watching people go through these trials, struggles, and losses. I've seen the suffering. I know how hard it's been.

Then one day, on top of it all, you stopped feeling well. Your energy started to flag, your jeans got harder to tug on, your heart started to race without prompting, your hair began to come out in clumps in the shower, you developed chills and hot flashes, your muscles began to ache, you stopped being able to concentrate, or your memory began to get fuzzy.

You may have had to resign from your job, quit classes, stop taking care of your kids as well as you'd like, said good-bye to friendships and opportunities, and despaired as your responsibilities fell by the wayside because it became a daily struggle simply to function.

The timing of your thyroid illness might have felt almost cruel. Just when life was feeling particularly difficult to balance, illness landed in your lap, throwing the very concept of balance out the window.

Or maybe your symptoms felt out of the blue. Everything was going along fine until suddenly, without warning, your life wasn't what it used to be. Suddenly, you weren't who you used to be.

In both of these cases—when illness feels like the last straw and when it feels like a sinkhole—we can understand how it got to this point through *triggers*. These are the events, emotional experiences, environmental factors, and other circumstances that can give the thyroid virus just the fuel it needs to go into an active growth state—in other words, to put you into a health crisis.

HOW TRIGGERS WORK

Once a person contracts the thyroid virus, its goal is to advance from the bloodstream to the lymph nodes to organs such as the liver to the thyroid to, ultimately, the central nervous system. During this process, there's often a bit of stop-and-start, which explains why you might have experienced better stretches of time and turns for the worse during your illness. At various points along the way, the virus will hide out in the body, building its numbers and waiting for the right moment to make its next move. And what determines those "right moments"? Triggers.

Do you remember the first time you stopped feeling like yourself, or the moment your previously manageable symptoms took a turn for the worse? Did it happen to come when you were experiencing intense financial worry, or after you'd gone through a divorce, other trauma, or given birth? These are just a few of the common triggers that can shift the thyroid virus from dormancy to attack mode and result in a thyroid problem—it's a bit like waking a grizzly bear from hibernation.

It's no coincidence that thyroid illness rears its head when you're already feeling off-kilter. That doesn't mean you attracted your illness with a stressed-out state of mind—not remotely. You didn't subconsciously will your body to break down by dwelling on negativity, either. Rather, intense experiences like these trigger off physiological responses—such as rushes of hormones, including excess adrenaline—that in turn give fuel to the virus. At the same time, these experiences and events signal the virus that the immune system isn't as strong as usual, meaning it's prime time for the virus to take advantage.

Then there are the triggers that have nothing to do with your emotional state. It could have been that you got a mouthful of metal fillings removed, releasing mercury (a favorite food of the thyroid virus) into your bloodstream. Or maybe you were exposed to another fuel of the thyroid virus, such as insecticides or pesticides, or an immune-system drainer, such as mold.

You'll hear from other sources that viruses simply self-replicate. If you've heard this, you've been misled. Regardless of what medical research and science have discovered so far, the truth is that viruses need fuel—whether in the form of hormones, toxins, or some of the actual foods that you eat (see Chapter 21, "Common Misconceptions and What to Avoid")—to reproduce.

While one trigger on its own can bring the thyroid virus out of dormancy, it's also common for several triggers to play a role, perhaps over years. Say, for example, your difficulty started in childhood, as you were taking on the stress of your parents or caregivers. As you grew older, maybe you went through a difficult relationship or two, got into a car accident, couldn't eat right, or lost sleep. These hardships, combined, took a toll on your body so that at certain points along the way, the thyroid virus—which you could have picked up at any point in life, from birth to school to a meal out just recently—saw opportunities to pounce.

THE TRIGGER LIST

As you read through the coming list of the most common thyroid virus triggers, see if any lightbulbs go off for you. Does the timing of your symptoms start to make sense with this new perspective?

Keep in mind that many of these triggers are ones you may have not been aware were present in your life at the time. You could have been exposed to pesticides without your knowledge, walked around with a nutritional deficiency that blood work didn't detect, or experienced another trigger, such as getting your carpets cleaned, that didn't register as a major life event.

As you think about these triggers, you may start to put the pieces together. Finally, you'll hold answers about why your illness struck at a certain time. The triggers are listed in order of prevalence, with the most common at the top and the less common ones at the bottom.

1. **Mold:** Prolonged exposure to mold in a building where you spend many hours of the day, such as a home or office, can wear away at your immune system, allowing the thyroid virus to take advantage.

2. **Mercury-based dental amalgam fillings:** If you have metal fillings (also called *silver fillings*), be careful about having them removed. The mercury they contain tends to be stable where it is, whereas the removal process can end up sending the toxic mercury into your bloodstream, giving food to the virus. If you want your metal fillings replaced, ask for them to be removed one at a time.

3. **Mercury in other forms:** Because mercury is one of the thyroid virus's favorite foods, avoid it in any form. For example, frequently eating seafood, especially large fish such as tuna and swordfish that tend to contain significant amounts of mercury, can eventually push your immune system past the breaking point and lead to infection of the thyroid virus. Mercury also tends to travel through bloodlines, contributing to health problems in generation after generation that are mistaken for genetic issues. Always be mindful about current mercury exposure, too—even in today's modern times, we're always vulnerable to coming into contact with it. Do your research, and question what's offered to you, your children, and the rest of your family.

4. **Zinc deficiency:** A zinc deficiency can also be inherited, and that deficiency can get worse over generations. If you're in a place in life where your zinc levels are particularly low, it can contribute to thyroid virus susceptibility.

5. **B_{12} deficiency:** Even if you get a blood test that shows your vitamin B_{12} levels are normal, that doesn't mean it's usable B_{12} that's absorbing where it needs to in your body. Your central nervous system, liver, or other organs may still be severely deficient, allowing the thyroid virus to grow rapidly.

6. **Pesticides and herbicides, including DDT:** Exposure to these poisons from sources such as sprayed lawns, gardens, parks, and golf courses can both damage your body and feed the thyroid virus with toxins that make it thrive. Pesticides and herbicides, especially DDT, can also be passed on from generation to generation—another inheritance that's often mistaken for a genetic issue.

7. **Insecticides in the home:** Flying bug spray, ant spray, roach spray, and other poisons meant to kill insects are poisonous for you, too. The toxins can build up in your organs, contributing to issues such as depression, and also fuel the thyroid virus.

8. **Death in the family:** Emotional trauma in any form can weaken

THE TRUTH ABOUT TRIGGERS

I hope that the simple act of reading this list has given you some insight into your particular circumstances. When you understand the why of your illness, it is a revelation that sets you on the true path to healing. When you eliminate that mystery about why sickness visited you at this time in your life, it puts the power back in your hands.

If you've been on the doctor shopping tour or read a lot about thyroid health, you might have learned already that experts suspect some of these factors are involved in thyroid illness—you might even have heard that some of the triggers you just read about are at the very root of thyroid illness. Let me be perfectly clear that these triggers are not to be mistaken for causes of thyroid virus symptoms. No matter what you've heard elsewhere, no matter which trigger, it is not the underlying reason you are sick. Further, these triggers do not put the blame on you. They don't make it so that somehow your sickness is your fault or the fault of the life you lead.

A trigger is only a trigger. One more time: *a trigger is only a trigger.* In order for it to give fuel to the thyroid virus, the virus has to be there in your system in the first place. (More on how easy it is to catch the virus in the next chapter.) Put it this way: The thyroid virus is like a fire. A thyroid virus trigger is simply gasoline thrown on the flames that makes them get hotter and spread faster.

This is why a husband and wife can both be exposed to mold—living, breathing, and even eating it in the same house every day—and the husband can be perfectly fine while the wife is bedridden from it, leaving both mold experts and health experts baffled. In that example, the wife has the thyroid virus in her system, and the mold is triggering it, while the husband is

virus-free. Or you could have a family of five exposed to mold on a daily basis, and only three family members come down with illness. Those three are the ones with the thyroid virus in their systems, and the mold has triggered the virus to become active and cause health problems. If everyone in the family gets sick, on the other hand, that's a sign that everyone has the thyroid virus. It's true that there are some varieties of mold so toxic that no one exposed to it will feel perfect. If one person (or more) exposed to this toxic mold in the home, office, car, or other source gets sicker than the rest, though, that usually indicates that this individual has the thyroid virus, and the mold wore down her or his immune system so the virus could take advantage.

While the virus I'm calling the "thyroid virus" sometimes comes up in medical discussions of thyroid problems, this incredibly common pathogen is not identified by medical communities as the *thyroid* virus. The virus is still considered secondary to thyroid illness; no one realizes the virus goes after the thyroid and causes all of the disruption there. Rather, observers have noticed that some people with thyroid issues also test positive for having been infected with the virus, and so they've made note that the two may be vaguely associated. Sometimes theorists guess that the virus is a trigger to autoimmune responses, which is not the case at all. *You* are the expert on the real triggers now.

While in many ways, it can be liberating to look at the trigger list, I understand that it may also feel overwhelming. After all, you can't control whether someone will break your heart or betray you. You can't make your loved ones live forever. You can't prevent all of life's injuries and accidents. Does that mean you're doomed to get sick every time one of these events crops up in your life?

Absolutely not. I don't want you to look at this list and feel afraid of life. Because here's the truth: We have a fundamental, God-given right to go through hardships unscathed. We're allowed to experience events that challenge us—we're *supposed* to go through these challenges—and they're not meant to bring us down. You have a fundamental right not to fear triggers. You are meant to have the freedom to experience life without illness.

So how do you move forward with this new knowledge? You use the information in the trigger list to heighten your awareness—so that you can protect yourself and your family from those triggers that *are* avoidable. And then, you take the measures you'll read about throughout this book to tame the thyroid virus, build up your immune system, and revive your thyroid—to take care of yourself the way you've always deserved, so that you're in prime shape to face all that life has in store for you.

CHAPTER 3

How the Thyroid Virus Works

Just how easy is it to catch the thyroid virus in the first place? Very. You could have picked it up from sharing a beer with a friend in college, from a kiss when dating, from eating out at a restaurant where an infected cook had a cut finger, from a blood transfusion, from sharing group bathrooms, from being sneezed on in elementary school—or you even could have gotten the virus at conception from your parents, because it's not uncommon for this virus to pass down through family lines.

While many of the early, crude varieties of the thyroid virus were more difficult to catch, and generally only transmitted through blood and occasionally saliva, the newer mutations of the thyroid virus (there are over 60 strains of it so far) are as easy to catch as cold or flu. Blood, saliva, tears, a runny nose, and more—intentional or unintentional exposure to these bodily fluids of someone who was in a contagious phase of the virus are all means of catching it. The virus is only a sneeze or a sip from a shared glass away.

And it is entirely possible that you could have picked it up without realizing at the time—because in its early stages, the thyroid virus

often doesn't cause any more symptoms than a brief and mild scratchy throat with some tiredness. Maybe there was a week or two, whether you were a child, teenager, or adult—or even when you were a baby—when you were feeling run-down for no identifiable reason, and then it passed. It could have seemed so unremarkable that you or your family didn't really register it, so the memory didn't stick.

Or maybe the virus made itself more than known after its incubation period, putting you through a month or more of extreme fatigue, feverishness, sore throat, headaches, swollen glands, and even rash—a memorable time of prolonged illness that eventually seemed to run its course.

In truth, even after any initial symptoms faded, the virus was making itself more and more at home in your body, moving along and building its numbers until one day, perhaps weeks or perhaps decades later—after the right triggers and circumstances converged—the virus could advance all the way to the thyroid, its best platform to get strong enough to inflame or go after your central nervous system.

WHAT IS THE THYROID VIRUS?

Some of the above information may sound familiar. A virus that's easy to pick up in college when sharing drinks and dorms, that's associated with kissing, and can give a person fatigue, fever, and sore throat for months . . . Does it sound like mono (a.k.a. glandular fever or "the kissing disease")? That's because it is.

That's right; the pathogen that I've been calling the "thyroid virus" is the same one that causes mononucleosis: *Epstein-Barr virus* (EBV). Medical communities have yet to discover that mono is only Stage Two of this virus—that in fact, the virus has four stages, the third of which targets the thyroid gland, explaining over 95 percent of thyroid problems. (The other 5 percent of thyroid problems come from radiation exposure due to chest, dental, and other X-rays; CT scans; food and water supply contamination; plane travel; cell phones; inheritance of our parents' and grandparents' exposure; and the continuous atmospheric radiation fallout from past nuclear disasters.)

EPSTEIN-BARR VIRUS TYPES

Epstein-Barr is a virus in the herpes family that has existed for well over 100 years. During that time, it has moved through many generations of people, mutating and elevating its various hybrids and strains along the way. Those strains—as I said earlier, there are over 60 of them—can be categorized into six groups of escalating severity, with roughly 10 types per group. Medical research and science have so far only found strains of the virus in one of those groups. When Anthony Epstein, Yvonne Barr, and Bert Achong reported their discovery of EBV in 1964,[1] they had most likely found what

I call Epstein-Barr virus numbers six and seven from Group 2. (This is not to be confused with the medical establishment's human herpesvirus numbering, which calls Epstein-Barr *HHV-4*. That term is merely the identification of the virus as a whole.) Soon after the landmark discovery of EBV, funding for further research was shut down, and that was all, folks. All these decades later, medical communities are as yet unaware that so many different groups and mutated strains of the virus exist.

Some strains of EBV (those in Group 1) are very mild and slow-moving; they may never result in anything more than a backache and may never progress as far as the thyroid. Other strains of EBV are more aggressive and fast-moving; they're responsible for some of the most debilitating illnesses of our time, including multiple sclerosis and various cancers. If you want to learn more about these EBV groups, I discuss them in more detail in the chapter "Epstein-Barr Virus, Chronic Fatigue Syndrome, and Fibromyalgia" of my first book, *Medical Medium*.

These various types of EBV explain why the virus presents so differently in different people. They also explain the wide range of thyroid issues out there. Goiters, for example, develop as a result of the first viral strain in Group 1. Hyperthyroidism and Graves' disease, on the other hand, are caused specifically by those varieties of EBV in Groups 4 and 5. These are aggressive strains that prompt the thyroid to produce extra thyroid tissue in self-defense, in turn causing the overproduction of thyroid hormones. EBV strains in Groups 4 and 5 also account for thyroid cancer (more on how thyroid cancer develops in Chapter 6, "Thyroid Cancer"). Benign tumors, nodules, and cysts, meanwhile, can be caused by EBV varieties from Groups 2 through 6. And Hashimoto's thyroiditis and hypothyroidism can be caused by any strain of EBV in any group.

Epstein-Barr virus is spreading at such an epidemic level right now that in 20 years, there will be close to 100 varieties—with most of the new ones hitting youth. It's bad enough that already roughly 17 out of 100 college students do not return to school after their first or second year due to the health effects of newer mutations of EBV. They're left back at home, lost and struggling with the virus's debilitating symptoms, many of them receiving Lyme disease diagnoses, which we'll cover later in this book. With no real answers about what's going on, these students despair as they try to figure out how they'll ever support themselves or live the lives they imagined. Now think about how many more children and young adults will be sidelined in two decades' time, with the virus's mutations progressing as they are.

It's why, more than ever before, this is a virus that needs our attention. It's why it's time for you to become an expert by reading this book. Knowing how the thyroid virus works is the only way to protect yourself and your loved ones from all the problems it has the potential to cause.

VIRAL POISONS

As you read about EBV's stages in the next section, there are a few terms it will be helpful to know. These are toxic castoffs that the virus creates as it replicates, and they usually cause problems in Stage Three (when the virus targets the thyroid) and Stage Four (when it goes after the central nervous system). They are a big part of what makes EBV so troublesome.

Viral byproduct: as EBV consumes its favorite foods, which include toxic heavy metals, excess adrenaline, and even eggs, if they're in your diet, it excretes this toxic waste matter. The more virus cells develop, the more byproduct is excreted and the more problems it causes, such as gumming up the mitral valve and creating heart palpitations.

Viral corpses: virus cells have a roughly six-week life cycle, which means that the cells are often dying off. These viral corpse cells are toxic, too, and as EBV grows in the body, there are more and more of them. You can think of viral corpses almost like dead crabs washed up on the beach, with shells (viral casings) that are either empty or still have some rotting meat inside. Because EBV cells shape-shift, these corpses end up with different shapes, as well. Viral corpse accumulation in the liver and lymphatic system creates sluggishness that often contributes to issues such as fatigue, weight gain, fluid retention, constipation, bloating, hot flashes, heart flutters, brain fog, and perimenopause/menopause symptoms. When someone has a lot of EBV activity in the body, the viral corpses eventually make it to the intestinal tract. If someone has a stool sample taken in this state, the hundreds or even thousands of viral corpses in the sample often confuse lab technicians and doctors, who mistakenly diagnose parasitical activity.

Neurotoxins: in later stages of the virus, EBV produces neurotoxins, poisons that disrupt nerve function. These neurotoxins come out as part of the virus's filmy byproduct sludge, then disperse, often inflaming the nerves and causing a great deal of pain. (Neurotoxins also reside in the viral corpses, if there's leftover "meat" inside their casings, and the neurotoxins can seep out as the corpses drift through the body.) These EBV excretions are made up of whatever the virus is feeding off of, such as mercury and other toxic heavy metals, and when these fuels "come out the other end" of the virus, they're even more corrupted versions of themselves—more disruptive and allergenic, almost like the venom of a poisonous spider or snake. EBV remanufactures these other toxins so that they become extra potent in their new form as viral neurotoxins, with a strength that can damage and kill off healthy cells in the organs and connective tissue. If the virus happens to consume excreted neurotoxins that it finds along the way the toxic materials are remanufactured again, and the potency of the poison is increased once more, able to do even more damage to cells as well as to irritate and inflame nerves with more intensity. EBV uses these poisons at strategic periods in Stage Three and continuously in Stage Four to prevent the immune system from zeroing in on the virus cells and attacking them.

Dermatoxins: similar to neurotoxins, these poisons are excreted by EBV when copper and pesticides such as DDT from generations past are sitting in the liver, giving a specific type of fuel to the virus. (As with neurotoxins, dermatoxins can also remain in viral corpses and seep out over time.) Because EBV tends to make the liver and lymphatic system sluggish and dysfunctional, they usually have trouble filtering out these poisons, so the toxins tend to escape through the skin, causing irritation, pain, itching, and/or rashes. These internal dermatoxins are much different from the known versions of dermatoxins, which are harmful chemicals that cause damage to the skin from the outside. EBV dermatoxins come from within, drifting up through the dermis, and they can result in someone receiving a diagnosis of eczema, psoriasis, or psoriatic arthritis. Because copper and DDT, like other toxins, can be passed down through generations, even the livers of newborns can contain them, which is how babies develop cases of eczema, psoriasis, and jaundice that baffle medical communities.

EPSTEIN-BARR VIRUS STAGES

As I said, EBV has four stages, and thyroid illness is what develops in Stage Three. Understanding all of the stages in more detail can help you better understand what you've been through—and what you want to prevent.

Stage One: The Baby Stage

When a person first catches EBV, or when someone is born with it, the virus is in the bloodstream, and it usually remains dormant. If you have EBV, then back at this early stage, it probably wouldn't have seemed like you were sick. The worst symptoms you might have experienced were listlessness, very mild fatigue, and a bit more susceptibility to colds, flus, sore throats, and earaches. For some people with mild cases of EBV, or those with robust immune systems, the virus will remain at this baby stage, dormant in the bloodstream and causing little to no discomfort, for the rest of their lives.

For those who've contracted more forceful strains of EBV that eventually cause thyroid problems and more, this is just the beginning. In these cases, the virus is quietly replicating in the blood, building its numbers for days, weeks, months, or many years, waiting for the right circumstances and the right trigger(s) so that it can develop into Stage Two: mononucleosis, followed by infection of organs such as the liver and spleen.

Luckily, it doesn't have to be this way. It's not inevitable that once contracted, the Epstein-Barr virus will march along to the organs and more. Here in Stage One, the virus is still vulnerable. If you know you've been exposed to someone in the contagious mono phase and you discover the antiviral measures in Part III, "Thyroid Resurrection," this is the point when it's easiest to get rid of most of the virus and to keep in check any that remains.

Stage Two: The War Stage

EBV often springs to life and enters Stage Two, which begins with mononucleosis, when someone has gotten particularly run-down. That's why college is such a prime time for students, who are up late partying and studying, and whose diet may have taken a turn for the worse since leaving home, to find themselves coming down with mono. Out of all the illnesses that sweep through colleges and universities, there isn't any more prevalent or rampant than mononucleosis—in other words, early Stage Two Epstein-Barr virus. It's unknown that 70 percent of all college students get mono sometime within their four years of school.

It's entirely possible to come down with mono before or after college, too. If you're dealing with a thyroid problem now and have no recollection of ever having had mono, consider the possibility that you went through it as a small child. Though nowadays, doctors are starting to diagnose mono in children as young as six, seven, or eight, traditionally, doctors only gave the "mono" label to older children. For the most part, it has been against the "rules" to diagnose mono in a child younger than six, regardless of what blood tests show. This is a classic regulatory issue in the medical field that holds back progress. In babies and young children, mono is and was often instead called "rheumatic fever" or "glandular fever," though it's really the same illness: Stage Two, active EBV infection.

Or you could have had mono as an adult and, if it was on the milder side, never realized what it was. Some people experience only a mild scratchy throat and some fatigue for a week; then it passes, and they never realize it was mono.

This phase is the point when the virus is infectious—if you have EBV, and it wasn't passed down your family line (meaning you've had it since birth), then you caught it from someone in your daily life who knowingly or unknowingly had mononucleosis. When you eventually reached your own mono phase, it could have been difficult for a doctor to diagnose. Blood testing for this is not completely reliable; it really comes down to each individual doctor's interpretation of either the antibodies that show up in your blood or subtle inconsistencies that aren't taught in medical school regarding the blood's white count. It's entirely possible that you simply never got the right label.

What's happening during mono is that your body's immune system is at war with the Epstein-Barr virus. At this point, instead of going stealth, as in Stage One when it wasn't causing any trouble, now the EBV starts releasing a chemical that announces to your immune system that an invader is present—it's like blowing the battle horn. EBV's goal here is to take down your lymphatic system, because that's your body's defense mechanism. Your immune system responds by sending identifier cells to "tag" virus cells with a hormone that marks them as invaders in your blood and lymph. Then it sends soldier cells to seek out and kill the tagged virus cells.

While this battle rages, a person experiences those mono symptoms, from mild to severe, depending on which viral strain or variety a person has. These symptoms, such as sore throat, fever, headache, and rash, are not signs of your body rebelling against you; they're actually signs of the power of your immune system coming to your defense. Sometimes these symptoms come and go. That's because at certain points, the immune system is able to get the virus under control; then it needs to gather its resources to fight the next battle.

At a certain point, the virus will get the message that it can't stay active forever, so it will begin looking for a long-term home in the body. Eventually, after just a week of mono or several months of it, the virus will pick an organ or organs, and it will recede from the bloodstream as it begins to nest. The war with the virus will die down, and EBV will enter Stage Two's second phase, when typically the virus is dormant and in retreat, though still alive and alert, camping out and lying in wait for triggers.

Unfortunately, this hiding-out mode doesn't stop the virus from causing problems. For everyone with Stage Two EBV—unless they're on a thorough antiviral protocol like the one you'll find later in this book—the virus ends up in the liver during this nesting phase. Why the liver? Because the liver is a filter for the body, so toxins such as mercury, dioxins, unhealthy fats, poisons that were passed down from earlier generations, and other waste matter accumulate there—and these just happen to be some of EBV's favorite foods to consume in order to stay alive and regenerate.

If you're trying to think back and understand how the virus might have affected you at this stage, ask yourself if there was any point at which you started to gain weight despite eating a healthy diet and exercising, or if there came a period when you started to feel more tired and listless than normal, possibly accompanied by a lack of motivation and a little brain fog. That's the likely time at which EBV got itself comfortable in the second phase of Stage Two. EBV and its toxic waste clog up the liver, making it sluggish, and a slowed-down, overloaded liver has everything to do with mysterious weight gain and changes in energy levels and mental clarity (more on these in Chapter 5).

Your doctor or trainer wouldn't have been able to tell you that EBV in the liver was the cause of the number going up on the scale, because current EBV tests are designed to detect the virus's presence in the bloodstream, not the organs. Instead, your doctor is likely to blame your weight gain on perimenopause or hormones or, if she or he keeps up with the latest theories, on your thyroid. Your trainer, meanwhile, might have blamed your weight gain on your exercise commitment or nighttime treats. Neither would have been right. It was never your fault.

Once EBV has moved on to the organs, those blood tests will indicate a *past* infection of EBV, not a present one. Medical training teaches that this means the virus is no longer causing problems. No one realizes that the virus has simply gone deeper into the body at this point, out of full battle mode, though alive and well on other levels and in other ways. This misinterpretation of EBV blood testing is how the virus has slipped through the cracks, preventing medical communities from understanding the full scope of EBV's harm. With all due respect, it's one of the greatest medical blunders of both history and our modern time.

What it will take for this to change is for more funding and research to go into interpreting lymphocyte, basophil, neutrophil, monocyte, and even blood platelet levels alongside EBV antibody levels—and to determine what the nuances of variations in these blood test results mean. Basically, an overhaul is needed in how professionals learn to read blood work. A "past infection" is probably very present and active somewhere in the body if these white blood cells show signs that they're putting up a fight. Is there something unusual going on with someone's lymphocytes, for example, while they also show "past infection" EBV antibodies? That's a good indication that EBV is at work in the organs and the reason for the patient's symptoms. Keep in mind that because blood work is still imperfect, as you'll read about in Chapter 6, "Thyroid Guess Tests," it's common to be living with EBV and for blood test results not to show anything amiss. Other times, though, it's there in the blood work for medical professionals to unlock. Is EBV about to move from the liver to the thyroid? Is it in the thyroid already, creating a nodule or hypothyroidism? Is it on its way to causing another illness from Chapter 5? In many cases, the markers are there. Only when medical communities see this can they get ahead of the EBV epidemic.

Other issues that can arise as a result of EBV nesting in the liver are an elevated A1C level; type 2 diabetes; high cholesterol; hepatitis A, B, C, and D; fibrosis; liver inflammation; development of sensitivities to foods that were never problematic before; and low hydrochloric acid in the stomach, the last of which translates to bloating, constipation, difficulty digesting food, and a toxic intestinal tract. This is often blamed on leaky gut syndrome, a misguided health theory that I talk about much more in *Medical Medium*.

For some people, the virus will hang out solely in the liver at this point. For many others, the virus will simultaneously burrow into the spleen and/or reproductive organs. EBV in the spleen (another filter for the body) will, over time, inflame the organ. The result is an enlarged spleen (splenomegaly) and spleen abnormalities that can give you a feeling of bloating or tenderness on your left side under your ribs.

When EBV goes to a woman's reproductive organs, meanwhile, it can lead to fibroids, polycystic ovarian syndrome (PCOS), and pregnancy complications. For men, one common target of EBV is the prostate, where the virus cells bury themselves and can, over a long period, result in cancer. That's right: EBV is the hidden cause of prostate cancer.

This nesting period of Stage Two can last from roughly one month to 20 years. It depends on what strain of the virus someone has, from which group, as well as on living conditions and exposure to triggers. For many people, EBV stays low-grade in the liver for decades, and may not move on to the next stage until someone is about age 50—especially if it's a milder variety of the virus. For others, EBV can progress from mono to liver infection to the next stage, thyroid infection, in as little as three months. A very common scenario is for nesting to last four to five years.

However long nesting lasts, the virus waits. Finally, when the right trigger or triggers come along—when someone goes through a time of profound grief or injury, for example, or an extra-large dosage of new medication, or anything else on the trigger list—the virus senses the excess stress hormones that go along with that immune system challenge. It identifies vulnerability and begins to take action, finally ready to make a break for its next target: the thyroid.

Stage Three: The Thyroid Stage

At this point, some people will experience what feels like another mild bout of mono. This won't show up as mono on blood tests, because you've already had mono once before, so doctors will most likely notice the antibodies indicating past infection and therefore determine that it can't be simultaneously active.

Meanwhile, the virus does become very active again, filling the liver with toxins that release into the lymphatic system and bloodstream and confuse the lymphocytes that protect the thyroid. These are lymphocytes specifically assigned to the thyroid area (and the tonsils, if need be). Medical research and science have not yet discovered that your thyroid has its own

tingles and numbness, thinning hair, brittle nails, dry skin, and dizziness. (For a much more extensive list, along with explanations of each, see Chapter 5.) These are all viral symptoms—some of them symptoms of the virus still living back in another organ—not thyroid-caused.

The immune system's priority during this ongoing battle is to protect the thyroid. If the virus has been in your thyroid for some time, then it's not uncommon for nodules (small lumps) to develop on the gland. These are calcium prisons the body creates to try to wall off the virus. Over time, if the trapped viral cells stay particularly active, the nodules can develop into cysts. Alternatively, sometimes small cysts develop on scar tissue in the thyroid—these can grow into benign tumors. And with those rare, aggressive varieties of EBV from Groups 4 and 5, cancerous tumors can develop in the thyroid—which is usually an indication that someone also has high levels of toxins in her or his organs.

The virus's aim in targeting the thyroid is to weaken your endocrine system. A compromised thyroid shifts the adrenals into overdrive, which can last for quite some time, and all that excess adrenaline is like a feast for the virus. EBV uses the adrenaline and cortisol to get bigger and stronger, and from this platform, it waits for just the right trigger (such as a heartbreak or divorce) or fuel (such as excess adrenaline or one too many egg-and-cheese sandwiches) to advance to its ultimate goal: the central nervous system. Not that this is inevitable—all of this can be stopped, reversed, or controlled before it develops further.

Stage Four: The Mystery Illness Stage

As with the transition from Stage Two to Stage Three, some virus cells stay behind causing trouble at this point, even as the virus cells on the front lines cause new trouble ahead. In other words, as the virus begins to affect a person neurologically, it will usually continue to damage the thyroid *plus* burden the organs it targeted back in Stage Two. Epstein-Barr can even move from Stage Three to Stage Four in as little as one day, meaning that it can begin to go after the thyroid and the central nervous system at almost the same time.

Luckily, many people never reach this stage. With the information in this book, you can keep a case of Stage One, Two, or Three EBV from reaching this most debilitating of stages. And if you have reached this stage, have no fear—you have the opportunity to get better. The battle can be won.

As more mutations make their way into the population, many more people, at younger and younger ages, will get here to Stage Four—if they don't have someone in their lives to share the truth revealed in these pages. So many people in their teens and early 20s are dealing with mystery symptoms such as fatigue, confusion, anxiety, depression, despondency, stomachaches, and racing thoughts. Sometimes these issues are ignored, sometimes they're chalked up to adolescent angst, and sometimes they're tagged with labels such as attention-deficit/hyperactivity disorder (ADHD), bipolar disorder, *Candida*, or depersonalization. Prescriptions often accompany these diagnoses, though they often don't help, because they're not addressing the true underlying viral issue. In a number of cases, young people are receiving misdiagnoses—what's really going on for so many of those who are suffering is Stage Four EBV getting underway.

With a misdiagnosis of ADHD, for example, what may really be going on for a given person is viral-caused brain fog and confusion that make it difficult to focus, alternating with racing thoughts and restlessness from EBV's neurotoxins. It's not ADHD "proper," which is mercury-caused. It's similar with misdiagnoses of bipolar disorder: someone may actually be experiencing periods of flatlining neurological fatigue and neurotoxin-induced depression alternating with periods of intense activity that occur when the virus has abated a bit, giving the person just enough energy that viral anxiety kicks up to throw them into a flurry. With *Candida*, it's frequently EBV and resulting liver dysfunction causing gut trouble, not this beneficial fungus, nor any parasites or the misunderstood "leaky gut." (For the explanation of true—not viral-caused—ADHD, what's really going on with *Candida* and digestive health, and more insight into depression, see the chapters devoted to them in *Medical Medium*.)

And with depersonalization, what shows on the surface of these young people is despondency, detachment, and thoughtlessness. What's so often going on *beneath* the surface is that EBV's neurotoxins are short-circuiting neurological communications, interfering with a brain that's still trying to develop. Because the brain isn't fully developed until well into a person's 20s, this result of Stage Four EBV is a widespread issue, making so many young people feel beyond isolated and their loved ones feel powerless to help. It's one of the disasters occurring in today's world—and entirely avoidable if the word about EBV gets out there.

No matter your age, if you're already dealing with one of these issues or with mystery illnesses such as fibromyalgia, chronic fatigue syndrome (CFS), rheumatoid arthritis (RA), tinnitus, vertigo, Ménière's disease, pulmonary fibrosis, cystic fibrosis, interstitial lung disease, Ehlers-Danlos syndrome, other connective tissue disorders, sarcoidosis, restless legs syndrome, or multiple sclerosis (MS), then you are already an expert on the disruption Stage Four EBV can cause in life—both physical and emotional.

Stage Four EBV is often the one that results the most in sufferers feeling or being told that they are crazy, lazy, liars, and/or delusional. Blood tests, X-rays, MRIs, and CT scans can't diagnose it, which leaves doctors massively confused about the droves of patients visiting them with mystery neurological symptoms. Family members and friends, too, may have a difficult time validating someone who can't offer a medical explanation about why she or he is unable to perform her or his normal functions. This is often the time when EBV sufferers feel most alone, knowing deep down that they would never make up the aches and pains, brain fog, dizziness, extreme fatigue, and more—and yet left to wonder if maybe they're deluding themselves, and they truly are making up their illness or causing it in some way.

Well, wonder no more. There is a very real, physical explanation for all of it. At Stage Four of EBV, viral neurotoxins flood the body's bloodstream and travel to the brain, where they short out neurotransmitters; plus the virus inflames or goes after the nerves throughout the body, making them sensitive and even allergic to the neurotoxins. As a result, it's common to experience heavier brain fog, memory loss, confusion, depression, anxiety, migraines, joint pain, nerve pain, heart palpitations, eye floaters, restless legs, ringing in the ears, insomnia, difficulty healing from injuries, and more. When you get to Chapter 5, you'll discover the particulars of these symptoms and conditions.

When nerves are injured, whether from an accident or by EBV, they send an "alarm" hormone to notify your body that the nerves are exposed and need repair. During Stage Four, EBV detects that hormone and rushes to the scene to latch onto the root hairs that hang off of the damaged nerves.

As the virus makes itself at home in or around the central nervous system, it inflames nerves. EBV's game plan with this is to slow down your body, so that your vascular system (blood vessels) can't deliver ample amounts of oxygen to your organs. Oxygen keeps the nervous system strong, plus it's an antiviral imperative to healing. When oxygen is not present in adequate amounts in the body, it creates a campground for EBV to grow and proliferate, also contributing to connective tissue disorders. This is why the trendy high-fat diets of today are detrimental to people with neurological symptoms and conditions—because the high fat level in the bloodstream diminishes oxygen levels, allowing for viruses to thrive.

In Stage Four, as in the other stages, EBV is always ready for that adrenalized moment in someone's life that will give it a surge of the stress hormones it loves. Any experience that induces a fight-or-flight, fear-factor type reaction—such as being in a car accident, receiving bad news, being emotionally attacked or backstabbed, going through a divorce or other traumatic breakup, or giving birth—is liable to act as fuel for Stage Four to progress even further.

If you experienced a fibro flare-up, for example, after you and your partner had a devastating fight, you may have come to believe that you manifested your illness from dwelling on the negative emotions surrounding the event. Don't let that thinking torture you for a moment longer. You can now understand your illness in a new, true light: After the trauma of that argument, if you went through a period of despair, grief, and depression that you couldn't shake off, you weren't failing to perk up and move on with life like a "normal" person, in this way making up your muscle pain and brain fog, or somehow creating them.

You were having a completely human, biologically hardwired response to trauma—which the virus wasn't helping, with its existing presence in your bloodstream and nervous system. Then, to make matters worse, when the viral symptoms hit you even harder than usual, that became its own trauma, not to mention a physical burden. (For more on hidden, everyday posttraumatic stress disorder, or PTSD, see the chapter devoted to it in *Medical Medium*.)

It's important for you to know that no matter what adrenalized events in your life may have brought on various flare-ups, you were not stuck in a vicious cycle of making yourself sick by perpetuating "negative" energy or thinking "wrong" thoughts. It was all physiologically explainable.

Flare-ups can also occur as part of the battle between your immune system and the virus. When you're killing off EBV in hard-to-reach places in your body, sometimes EBV will try to balance its loss by sending out another proliferation, starting second or third cycles of the virus that bring back your frustrating symptoms.

Very often, doctors mistake Stage Four EBV for adrenal fatigue. While adrenal fatigue does exist, and it can be very challenging (I devoted a chapter to it, too, in my first book), medical communities do not yet realize what the true missing piece is. No matter what you hear elsewhere about how prevalent adrenal fatigue is, it is not the be-all, end-all health insight you may be led to believe. Adrenal fatigue (or thyroid problems, for that matter) as the explanation of the world's problems is not accurate.

What's really behind the worst, life-limiting exhaustion is *neurological* fatigue—and that's a symptom of Stage Four EBV that we'll explore in more detail later in this book, along with the other symptoms and conditions that EBV causes. It's a symptom medical research is only at the very beginning of identifying on a surface level.

Medical communities don't yet have a sense of neurological fatigue's cause or scope or its tie to late-stage EBV—not least because medical communities don't yet realize there *is* late-stage EBV. This neurological fatigue is the number one reason those roughly 17 out of 100 college students with EBV can't return to school—and in many cases can't return to any normal life, because they're struggling to survive.

Stage Four EBV is not a life sentence. When you learn the true cause of what's keeping you ill, and when you learn to use the tools contained in this book about how to resurrect your health, you hold the power to rebuild your immune system and regain control. It's not solely about getting back your liver or your reproductive system or your thyroid or your nervous system—it's about getting back your life.

THE AUTOIMMUNE LINK

So let's recap: It's not your own immune system that's responsible for hypothyroidism (underactive thyroid), hyperthyroidism (overactive thyroid), thyroiditis (inflammation of the thyroid), or nodules, tumors, cysts, and tissue damage to the thyroid gland. It's the thyroid virus—EBV—at an advanced stage. It's not even your own immune system that's causing the autoimmune-labeled Hashimoto's thyroiditis or Graves' disease. Again, it's the virus that's responsible. Your immune system is on your side. Knowing this is critical to your healing. It is one of the most important factors in getting better.

The Epstein-Barr virus doesn't just explain "autoimmune" diseases of the thyroid. EBV is behind a number of other autoimmune disorders, too. If you've ever worried that because of a diagnosis of Hashimoto's or Graves', you have a tendency toward autoimmunity in general, and are therefore in more danger of developing additional autoimmune illnesses—or if you've already developed other autoimmune conditions alongside Hashimoto's or Graves'—set your mind at ease. It is extremely likely that your other issues come from the same source as the thyroid problems: the virus. This means that even though you may have ten symptoms or illness labels, you probably don't have ten separate diseases—it may only be this one thing, EBV, that's wrong. Addressing that could take care of it all. This is another critical piece of knowledge as you work on healing.

Epstein-Barr is responsible for an overwhelming number of so-called autoimmune conditions, including CFS; fibromyalgia; eczema and psoriasis; psoriatic arthritis; hepatitis A, B, C, and D; MS; RA; and lupus. These conditions have nothing to do with a faulty body; they have everything to do with the immune system putting up the fight of its life against this invader. In Chapter 5, we'll look at some of these illnesses in more detail. For now, know that to understand EBV is to understand autoimmunity. Everything you'll read in this book will shed light on that.

And everything you'll read in the chapters to come will help you better understand where you are now and how to move forward into a better, more promising future. That begins with coming to appreciate your thyroid for its true and undiscovered capabilities.

CHAPTER 4

Your Thyroid's True Purpose

This small gland in the front of your neck is not the metabolism manager everyone thinks it is. The thyroid hormones that have been discovered so far—and the ones yet to be discovered—do not directly control your weight or regulate your hunger or ignite your libido or elevate your energy. This concept of metabolism is oversimplified and outdated. *Metabolism* is simply a name for the antiquated discovery that the body is in a constant state of internal change and movement. It's the discovery that we're alive. It's one of those blanket terms that obscures the fact that so much is not yet known about it.

Your thyroid's true function and purpose is actually much more interesting than the modern medical understanding of it. Truth is, your thyroid is your body's data center. *It is your second brain.* And here's the kicker: Even when it's been damaged by the Epstein-Barr virus or surgically removed, your thyroid can still do this main job. And since the rest of the endocrine system is so advanced, too, it can fill in for the rest.

As the data center, your thyroid catalogues all the markers of homeostasis in your body. (Homeostasis is the state of physiological equilibrium among your various body systems—it means everything when it comes to your health.) Your thyroid records what balance looks, feels,

and acts like for you individually. Messages from every organ and every gland get delivered to the thyroid—when necessary, as complaints. Like a human resources department in a company, your thyroid fields these reports, collecting and recording data about what's functioning well in your body, what's not functioning, what's toxic, and what's not toxic.

Then, day in and day out, your thyroid uses its memory of homeostasis to send out radio-like frequencies (not yet detected or measured by medical science or research) that delegate tasks and responsibilities throughout the body to keep everything in balance. Your thyroid, which is self-powered and self-sufficient, uses its intelligence about your personal homeostasis to continuously re-create it for you, so that when one body system is overtaxed or compromised, another kicks in to compensate. As the thyroid delivers different frequencies to different parts of the body as needed, it can even provide energy to them—energy that is not yet weighed or measured by research and science.

For example, when the liver is losing strength due to an illness, the pancreas has to work harder. The thyroid picks up this message, and sends extra radio-like frequencies to the liver to recalibrate and support it, at the same time giving the pancreas extra energy for support.

Even when the thyroid itself is compromised, it can still perform these vital functions.

THYROID HORMONES

Out of all the thyroid does, its least important task is its production of the hormones thyroxine (T4) and triiodothyronine (T3). Remember, medical research and science only theorize about the impact of T4 and T3 on health. The functions of these hormones can't be weighed or measured in any lab or study yet. T4 and T3's physical purpose is still a medical mystery, and no one's allowed to admit or dispute that. It's another theory held as truth and law, and the door to exploring it is closed—what I call a *closed-door theory*. While medical communities so far believe this hormone production to be the most important function of the thyroid—theorizing that these hormones have a role in the metabolism of every cell—this is not the case. Yes, the thyroid has a role in regulating all of your cells through its work to promote homeostasis—though that doesn't completely hinge on T4 or T3.

The known thyroid hormones are not the most significant. Think about it: If the underproduction of thyroid hormones were truly the defining aspect of so many thyroid illnesses, then why wouldn't the illness go away when someone went on hormone replacement medication? Ask the millions of women on thyroid medication if, since starting the hormones, they no longer struggle with weight gain, hair loss, feverishness, insomnia, and so on down the list. Some of them may have felt some improvement on medication—in most cases because they overhauled their diet and exercise programs

at the same time. However, an overwhelming number of these people will say that their symptoms have not vanished. That's because these symptoms are viral, not hormonal, so hormones don't fix them.

T4 and T3 do play a role in your health. Science is unaware that their true functions are to keep the immune system balanced to prevent under- or overreaction to stimulus, to help keep body temperature level, and to support the pancreas. Very few actual symptoms occur when the thyroid is not producing enough of these two hormones, though.

Essentially, T4 and T3 are steroid compounds, and when the thyroid is underactive and weakens, your body has built-in mechanisms to compensate for that loss. Your thyroid places a 911 call to the rest of the endocrine system and other organs for backup. To begin with, a healthy, functioning liver will have a "storage bin" of T4—which it can also convert to T3—so it will release these hormones if the thyroid is underactive and distressed. In fact, T4-to-T3 conversion in the first place is much more of a liver function than a thyroid one. If you've heard that you have a conversion problem, know that this has to do with your liver—it's probably become overburdened from the EBV, combined with other toxins such as pesticides and heavy metals or prescription medications. A dysfunctional liver is the true cause of thyroid hormone conversion problems.

If your liver is compromised due to the EBV or other factors, your pancreas will increase its release of the hormone insulin in order to help convert T4 to T3, as well as its enzyme output to elevate the digestive process. Plus, your adrenals will step in with their own tailor-made steroid blend to help replace and mimic the diminished thyroid hormones. (This adrenaline blend won't be detected as thyroid hormone on blood tests because it's subtly different in composition. Since no one is aware that the body has this hormone replacement system, blood work isn't designed to detect it, and it stays off the radar.) The end result is that you're mostly protected from feeling the effects of lower thyroid hormone production.

The thyroid-related hormones known as thyroid-stimulating hormone (TSH) and thyrotropin-releasing hormone (TRH) do also play their own roles—and the body also has powerful ways of filling in for them when anything goes awry. TSH is the bell at the schoolhouse telling everyone to get to class. Produced by the pituitary gland, its job is to notify the thyroid in turn to produce T4 and T3. And TRH from the hypothalamus is what tells the pituitary to release its hormone in the first place.

The hypothalamus is your body's safety mechanism in this case. If something happens to harm the pituitary, the hypothalamus can actually mimic TSH, calling for the thyroid to produce T4 and T3. It's yet one more of the body's backup, standby, failover systems. In rare cases, the Epstein-Barr virus will attack the hypothalamus, interrupting this process, though that's rare.

What *is* most important about how the thyroid works is its function as institutional memory and peacekeeper among all the organs and glands—and this doesn't require T4 or T3 or its signalers TRH or TSH. Rather, the thyroid produces two additional thyroid hormones that are not yet discovered by medical research and science: I call them R5 and R6. (There's a good chance research will name them this, too, though if given another name, they will be the same hormones.) These play a pivotal role in the radio-like frequencies that the thyroid emits in its messaging and monitoring of the body.

Yet more safety measures are in place here: These hormones are virtually impossible to deplete, plus the liver keeps a storage bin of them as backup. And as with the other thyroid hormones, the adrenals can produce adrenaline blends that mimic R5 and R6 when needed.

We tend to hold on to what we know and make that the focus. It's much like how sunlight provides us with a whole range of health benefits, and yet vitamin D alone gets the attention. The medical fixation on current thyroid medications plus the known hormones T4, T3, TSH, and TRH will one day subside as new research comes to light about additional thyroid hormones and the thyroid's true, primary function in your body. Right now, we're still at, "Here, take this pig or synthetic thyroid, and go off on your way." That's as far as we've come in over 100 years. Someday, medical research will put together the missing pieces of the thyroid's true purpose in the body. In the meantime, *you* know, and that's critical to your healing.

THE ADRENAL LINK

Now back to the thyroid virus. What does all of the above mean in relation to EBV? That you are remarkably resilient. Despite all of the disruption that the virus tries to create by targeting the thyroid, it cannot take it down. Your thyroid and the backup systems that support it are too advanced for EBV. Even if your thyroid isn't there because the virus has damaged it so much that you had it surgically removed or "killed off" with radioactive iodine, it can still do its job, as you'll read more about in Chapter 19, "Time to Rebuild Your Body."

Now, all this compensating that the body has to do when EBV goes after the thyroid does create some issues elsewhere. To begin with,

EBV's attack jolts the immune system, then starts to drain it. This is one of EBV's goals: to try to disrupt homeostasis and throw off the immune system.

And when the thyroid is under-producing hormones, the adrenal glands (the most important part of the endocrine system) need to squeeze out the replacement steroid I mentioned earlier. This is a truly remarkable process: Think of the adrenals as the most advanced chef or chemist on the planet, one who can formulate an exact recipe to mimic a missing ingredient. It's truly remarkable—these faux thyroid hormones are actually shape-shifting chemicals that fill in for exactly what your body needs. This is why people can walk around with a hypothyroid and not experience a single symptom—not even from the underlying EBV. The adrenals are both compensating for the low thyroid hormones *and* giving you extra juice to function as the virus tries to drain you. Regardless of how battered or fatigued your adrenal glands get, they will always compensate for your thyroid. This mechanism is built in to the human body, and the only factor that can get in

the way is if something terrible happens to your adrenals, and you lose them altogether.

This process of adrenal compensation is completely necessary. Without it, you wouldn't be able to function. The downside is that, as I've mentioned before, the Epstein-Barr virus loves all that extra adrenaline; it's one of its favorite foods. So even as your body does a miraculous job of keeping itself balanced so that you can get through each day, EBV isn't ready to call it quits. It's still hungry, and it still has its sights on your central nervous system—unless you know how to stop it.

An important step in understanding EBV well enough to put an end to it is discovering the how and why of your specific symptoms and conditions. Now that you know about the triggers for EBV, its types and stages, and just how powerful your thyroid and the systems that support it are—now that you see that your thyroid was never behind your illness—it's time for you to see the particulars of how the virus has been behind your symptoms and conditions all along. You're about to discover one of the most important elements of how to finally heal.

CHAPTER 5

Your Symptoms and Conditions—Explained

In the late 1800s, the Epstein-Barr virus was still very mild. The pathogen wasn't terribly contagious or aggressive then; it took a direct exchange of bodily fluids with someone who was experiencing an active EBV infection to catch it—and those active infections were somewhat rare. EBV could live dormant in someone for an entire lifetime without causing problems or symptoms.

That's because EBV got its start as a productive virus. Medical science has only begun to document the possibility that beneficial viruses exist. In the future, researchers will find that it's much more than a possibility—it's reality. That's right: Just like we have "good" bacteria that help protect our health, "good" viruses exist, as well. These are docile, beneficial bugs we carry around that help keep our immune systems in gear. EBV used to be one of them. In its most elementary, fundamental state, EBV was a gentle bug that was on our side and did no harm. In fact, it even helped remove toxic waste from our bodies. Before the late 1700s, the waste in our systems was mainly a byproduct of natural bodily functions; the rest of it came from food we consumed and some heavy metals in their

early, unaltered forms. EBV was our friend, scavenging for toxins throughout the body, including in and around the liver, spleen, intestinal tract, lymphatic system, and even bloodstream, so they wouldn't harm us. Then EBV went over to the dark side—though it wasn't the virus's fault.

Two waves of modernization turned EBV into what it is today. First came the Industrial Revolution. In the late 1700s and early 1800s, when mankind began to manipulate chemical compounds like never before, employing toxic heavy metals in new ways, generating potent chemical reactions, then burning and disposing of the compounds, various pollutants made it into our air and waterways. As these toxins got into people's systems, EBV was given new foods. The virus was still docile and beneficial, scavenging for the toxins to protect us, however these new Industrial Revolution toxins slightly poisoned the virus. In order to protect *itself*, the virus would excrete them—in more toxic form, because the viral processing increased their potency. EBV cells would enter a cycle of re-consuming these poisons, and it became survival of the fittest. The EBV cells that were able to withstand the processed and re-processed poisons survived and multiplied, and the weaker virus cells died off. While still trying to be on our side, EBV needed to look out for itself now, too, and it became stronger than ever.

Then in the late 1800s and early 1900s, a wave of experimental fungicides, herbicides, and antibiotics (ones that predated the penicillin discovery and boom) were created. These concoctions contained risky ingredients such as arsenic, copper, lead, and petroleum; early, crude chemical compounds newly synthesized in labs for industrial use; plus fungus and mold grown on petroleum waste from the oil and gas industry, and they were just the right fuel to bring EBV to life. Some of the crude antibiotics made it into early pharmacy drugs. You never learned about this in history class or medical school, because it isn't public knowledge that it took decades of reckless, failed lab experiments with toxic ingredients to lead to the eventual discovery of penicillin. Barrels of dangerous brews were also dropped off for free at farms across the country, rather than sold in stores or advertised in magazines. Though this remains undocumented, it was the advent of spraying down every piece of food in the field. (This was long before the Green Revolution of conventional food growing; this unknown chemical era predates even the early research and development phase of the Green Revolution by 50 years.)

People's exposure to these concoctions, however hidden, was widespread—their food, medicine, and water supplies became contaminated, and as a result, any EBV in their systems got what it needed to grow in leaps and bounds, and with it, other bugs, too, such as the first variety of EBV's cofactor, *Streptococcus* bacteria. In other words, these dangerous brews gave the virus just what it needed to "hulk out" and go to war with the immune system, initiating the first cases of glandular fever. Suddenly, not only

were individual cases of EBV transforming from harmless to problematic as EBV developed a palate for industrialized, lab-developed chemicals; now the amped-up, mutating virus was moving across the population at a much faster rate. Like a friend turned against us, EBV had become an enemy.

It took decades for the effects of this shift to become apparent on a widespread scale. Because of EBV's stop-and-start tactic, where it can spend years dormant and silently multiplying while it waits for the perfect trigger to make its next move, the length of time it took these early unproductive EBV strains to showcase themselves was considerable. A few cases of thyroids swollen by still-mild EBV combined with iodine deficiency resulted in the identification of Hashimoto's thyroiditis in the early 1900s (not that doctors identified EBV as the cause). Then it wasn't until the early 1940s that the first surge of people began to come down with the hot flashes, aches and pains, brain fog, mystery infertility, hair loss, and excessive fatigue so typical of EBV when it wakens from dormancy. By about 1950, EBV symptoms had reached an epidemic level—what I call *epic-demic* for the massive effect on society and public health. The people suffering were ones who had been born in the late 1800s and early 1900s, as EBV was gaining momentum in the population. Now they were feeling its effects without knowing the true cause.

In droves, women were visiting the doctor for answers. And yet medical research and science didn't have the diagnostic tools or framework to explain to themselves or their patients what was going on. It was a frightening time. No one could understand why so many middle-aged women were suddenly feeling so unwell—and so it was the birth of "crazy women syndrome" and "It's all in your head," echoes of the "hysteria" label women had received for thousands of years.

As women's mystery symptoms continued to build and progress, though, it wasn't quite as easy to pass off this suffering as laziness or an overactive imagination. Coincidentally, pharmaceutical science had been focusing on hormone research at the time, and so experts started to connect the two. In some women, they mistakenly diagnosed EBV symptoms as a hormone imbalance from menopause. In others, they mistakenly diagnosed those same symptoms as a thyroid hormone imbalance. Some women received both diagnoses.

Still, since these weren't the real answers, the treatments didn't make people better. Through the decades, mystery symptoms in the population continued to build, with new labels entering the scene to try and make sense of it: multiple sclerosis, perimenopause, Lyme disease, chronic fatigue syndrome, fibromyalgia, even "yuppie syndrome." Now experts in chronic illness are trying to crack the case by saying that the thyroid has been the problem everyone's looking for. It's not. All along, it's been the Epstein-Barr virus.

In most cases, a doctor won't be able to identify EBV as the problem, because the most advanced medical information out there still says that if a test doesn't detect active EBV in your bloodstream, then the virus is not to blame for your ills. Even if EBV is detected, the likelihood is that it still won't be identified as the source of your health issues, because medical communities haven't learned yet what an EBV symptom is. The furthest they've gotten is to identify mono's flu-like symptoms such as fatigue, fever, and swollen glands. They don't have a checklist of all those EBV symptoms that come *after* EBV's mono stage, because they don't realize there are symptoms after mono.

They have no idea that your health issues are related to this virus.

It's very common to hear that your blood-test results show antibodies that indicate a *past* infection of EBV, and that the virus therefore isn't an issue anymore. Don't let this mislead you. EBV tests simply aren't advanced enough yet to detect the virus once it's moved on from mono. (For more on this, see Chapter 7, "Thyroid Guess Tests.") And as you read about in Chapter 3, "How the Thyroid Virus Works," it's after the mono phase that the virus really starts causing trouble.

Yes, the thyroid illness epidemic is real— across the country and the world, people's thyroids are compromised. This doesn't explain why these people are suffering, though. It doesn't explain the multitude of symptoms that are causing people to lead diminished lives. Rather, a thyroid issue is one big, giant arrow to the much larger source problem: EBV. The thyroid is the victim in the situation, wrongly blamed.

You can think of it like a clown performing at a birthday party, popping balloon after balloon in children's faces. As the kids start to cry at the *pop* after *pop*, it becomes a circus gone wrong, when all you wanted was a clown with a happy face to make some funny balloon art. What is this, a mean clown? It thinks it's funny to upset the kids? Our instinct is to fault the clown, withhold pay, and send it packing. We're wary of clowns to begin with, not quite sure what their deal is beneath the surface, and we forget there's a human being inside the costume. It's just like how we're taught to be wary of our bodies—our thyroids in particular—thinking they could turn on us at any moment, without giving enough credit to the soul inside. If we did a thorough investigation of the clown incident, we'd find that she was doing everything right, just trying to please her young crowd, and it was the balloon factory's supplier that was at fault. The factory had gotten in a bad batch of latex, and it hadn't just affected her balloon animals. That supplier's contaminated latex was causing issues in all sorts of products across the globe—it was a sign of a much bigger problem.

EBV is like that tainted batch of latex, the real cause of that three-ring thyroid circus. If people knew that it wasn't the thyroid's fault, they'd have a much different perspective on the wonders of their bodies and their prospects for healing. Instead of hating their thyroids, they'd treasure them.

This is critical information for you to hold close, because modern-day medical explanations of hormonal imbalance and thyroid disease leave countless people feeling that their bodies aren't to be trusted. It's also very common for thyroid patients to suffer from multiple health issues, and to think that this means that there's something wrong with them at the core, because they haven't yet discovered that EBV is at the root of all of it. They feel betrayed, defective, weak—when in fact, it's just the opposite. Your body fights for you. Your body is on your side. Your body loves you unconditionally. It happens to be up against a pernicious adversary in EBV—though it's one that can be tamed with the approach you'll find in this book.

Connecting to this truth and all of the knowledge you've gained so far about what thyroid illness really is, how it came to be, and how it works is a tremendous step in healing from any thyroid condition and its related issues. You didn't cause your illness. Your body's not letting you down. You're not to blame. You can move forward. You can heal.

WHAT YOUR SYMPTOMS MEAN

As I've said, thyroid issues themselves are not symptomatic to the degree experts think; they are not, in fact, the problem. They're only a signal, a clue—a puzzle piece to the much bigger picture that is EBV. For that reason, in the list to come, all of the labels for thyroid illnesses are included as *symptoms* of this thyroid virus. This may seem surprising at first. As you take in the information, you'll see why it makes sense.

In this list, you'll also find those health problems more commonly known as symptoms, such as memory loss, body temperature fluctuations, chills, night sweats, and heart palpitations. As you'll see, these are nearly always symptoms of EBV. Though some of them can have other explanations (for example, muscle cramps can also occur as a result of nutrient deficiencies, or you may get a mild fever from severe dehydration), if you've come to this book with a thyroid issue or you experience multiple issues on this list, there's a good chance that the given explanation for a symptom below describes what's going on for you. Before reading on, there's something important to keep in mind: What you find here won't be misinformed theories or standard explanations with non-useful information. You're about to enter new territory regarding what causes a given symptom or condition.

Hypothyroidism

Hypothyroidism is a mild, early-stage case of thyroiditis. With EBV drilling into thyroid tissue, the gland becomes damaged and scarred, which impedes its function. In this weakened state—also called underactive thyroid or low thyroid—the thyroid can become less effective at producing its thyroid hormones T4 and T3. Hypothyroidism can cause body temperature fluctuations, a bit of fatigue or slight listlessness, and dry skin—that's it. What about all the other symptoms typically associated with low thyroid hormone levels? They're symptoms of the EBV wreaking havoc inside the liver and other areas of the body while also infecting the thyroid, not symptomatic of low levels of thyroid hormones.

Even congenital hypothyroidism, when a baby is born with an underactive thyroid, is from EBV. While developing in the womb, a baby is susceptible like we are, and a mutated strain of the virus can get into the baby's liver and eventually its thyroid, causing thyroid issues from birth.

Hypothyroidism would be a little more disruptive if not for your adrenals. As we looked at in the previous chapter, medical research and science have not yet discovered that your adrenal glands produce a hormone blend to compensate for the reduced T4 and T3—a blend that's almost exactly like your thyroid hormones, though just different enough that those few symptoms I just mentioned can sneak in. If the adrenals didn't perform this teamwork, the low T4 levels from your hypothyroid would cause inconsistent menstrual periods, a lack of motivation, higher levels of listlessness, and feelings of sadness—which are still not the "classic" symptoms that are (incorrectly) associated with hypothyroidism. Again, those "classic" symptoms are viral or viral-related.

When you have a hypothyroid, it doesn't automatically mean the whole gland is kaput. Much of the thyroid is still working beautifully. It would take true injury to the thyroid that completely disrupted and disassembled its inner workings to really take it down. You may think this describes you. If so, keep in mind that it is a *very* rare few for whom a hypothyroid itself is

the cause of any real symptoms. It would take a combination of physical injury to the thyroid (think strangulation or a severe blow to the throat), trust issues of the greatest magnitude, tragic loss in life, and mountains of stress to break down the spirit of the thyroid. (If you are one of those extremely rare few, take heart that you can still recover.) For the vast majority of people, the thyroid, no matter how damaged, is able to continue to do its job monitoring the body; plus the rest of the body is able to step in and compensate for its low hormone production, and the result is that any symptoms you feel are viral.

Hyperthyroidism and Graves' Disease

In some cases, instead of causing an underproduction of thyroid hormones, EBV prompts the thyroid to overproduce them. This is called hyperthyroidism—and the diagnosis that many people with hyperthyroidism receive is Graves' disease, an illness tagged as autoimmune that leaves far too many patients feeling that their bodies have let them down. This couldn't be further from the truth. Graves' disease is not a result of the immune system becoming confused and attacking the thyroid.

Rather, Graves' disease and hyperthyroidism occur because a particular strain of EBV—one that's a bit more aggressive and fast-moving than the strains behind hypothyroidism—causes an assault on the thyroid, which prompts the gland to overcompensate by rapidly creating new cells and tissue. This extra thyroid tissue produces extra thyroid hormones, resulting in the symptoms of bulging eyes, enlarged thyroid, swelling in the throat, a bit of fatigue, and temperature fluctuations. As with hypothyroidism, most of the symptoms associated with Graves' (such as sweating, high blood pressure, and nervousness) are virus-related and not a direct result of an overactive thyroid.

Though less common, it is possible to get a diagnosis of hyperthyroidism alongside Hashimoto's rather than Graves'. That's because a person can harbor two varieties of EBV at the same time, one of them accelerating cell and tissue growth, while the other is destructive toward thyroid tissue. This can easily result in widely fluctuating thyroid hormone readings, because one strain of the virus may be more active in a person's system at any given time, changing whether the thyroid is under- or overproducing hormones.

Inflammation, Enlarged Thyroid, and Hashimoto's Thyroiditis

When EBV targets the thyroid gland, the immune system reacts in full force, and the result is inflammation. Inflammation is the body's natural response to invasion and/or injury. Have you ever gotten a splinter, and soon the skin around it became red, hot, and puffy? That's the body responding with inflammation to a foreign object (invasion) that's causing cell damage (injury). The same goes for the thyroid. If EBV enters your thyroid tissue, your immune system immediately knows that it's present (invasion) and causing cell damage (injury), so the gland becomes inflamed. This can come with the feeling of a sore throat, pressure in the throat, or a funny feeling in your neck. It can also result in an enlarged thyroid. Further, you could have an inflamed thyroid with no symptoms at all, because everyone's different, and every case of inflammation is different. It all depends on which part of your thyroid is inflamed—whether

front, back, top, bottom, or on either side—and how inflamed it is.

If you've been diagnosed with thyroiditis, understand that it's a sign of your immune system working hard for you, doing everything in its power to fight the virus; it's not a malfunction of your body. The inflammation is not occurring because "autoantibodies" are being produced by your immune system to go after your own cell tissue. The antibodies that show up on thyroid tests are present because there's a battle going on in your thyroid between EBV cells and your immune system. That is, your immune system is producing the antibodies to seek out and destroy the Epstein-Barr virus that's causing thyroid damage or inflammation.

Let's think about the name "Hashimoto's thyroiditis" for a moment. While it may seem big and frightening and cast a shadow over your life, if you break it down, it will lose some of its power over you. *Thyroiditis*, first of all, means inflammation of the thyroid—that's it. And *Hashimoto* is nothing more than the name of the doctor who first identified swelling in his patients' thyroids. While this was a landmark discovery at the time, it was not a grand revelation about what was behind the inflammation. Rather, it was a doctor feeling his patients' necks, identifying thyroid swelling by touch, recognizing that iodine deficiency didn't wholly explain the problem, and saying, "Something's wrong here"—though not identifying what. The label only named the symptom of inflammation, not the underlying cause. As I mentioned at the beginning of the chapter, these initial Hashimoto's cases were in fact the earliest cases of EBV (after it had morphed into a destructive version of itself) taking advantage of iodine deficiencies and weak immune systems. When "Hashimoto's" starts to sound like an intimidating label, remind yourself that the discovery took place over a century ago. Now it's time to take the next step and uncover the answers.

It wasn't until the publication of my first book, *Medical Medium: Secrets Behind Chronic and Mystery Illness and How to Finally Heal*, which includes a chapter on hypothyroidism and Hashimoto's, that the truth finally reached the public about EBV as that real, underlying cause. It's time to reclaim your power and understand that Hashimoto's is a label and not a judgment or life sentence. The reason for your suffering does not come from within. Your immune system is not going haywire or out to get you. It's this virus—this invader—that's causing the damage, making you feel miserable, and holding you back in life. Your body just needs the proper support, which I describe in this book, to triumph over the virus.

Thyroid Nodules, Cysts, and Tumors

If you've ever been diagnosed with a thyroid nodule or cyst, you've probably found the diagnosis a bit unsettling. After all, none of us wants to hear that we have a growth, much less one that appears mysteriously with no answer about how to make it go away. Here's the truth about these lumps: they are yet another sign of your body working hard against the Epstein-Barr virus.

When the immune system isn't able to destroy the virus altogether, it goes with its fallback option: attempting to wall off the virus with calcium. That's what thyroid nodules are: calcium prisons for EBV cells. Unfortunately, this doesn't get rid of the virus, because (1) most of the EBV cells evade getting walled off, and (2) those EBV cells that do get trapped make themselves at home within the calcium walls, continuing to feed off the thyroid and drain it

of energy. If the virus cells prosper too much in the nodule, they can transform it into a living growth—a cyst—which puts even more strain on the thyroid. It's also possible to get a keloid scar on the thyroid, though doctors won't identify it as such. These keloids form when EBV creates extra tissue at the site of an injury to the thyroid, whether from outside impact or the virus itself.

If you've experienced larger thyroid tumors that are cancerous, know that these are caused by rare, particular strains of EBV. Their formation usually indicates that a person also has toxins such as elevated heavy metals and pesticides in her or his organs. (For more on thyroid cancer, see Chapter 6.)

Meanwhile, all that calcium walling off the virus has to come from somewhere. If a person with a thyroid nodule or cyst doesn't have enough calcium in the bloodstream because she or he isn't eating enough calcium-rich foods, then the immune system will extract calcium from the bones, which can lead to osteopenia and eventually osteoporosis. Do not be misled when you hear that thyroid issues *cause* osteoporosis. When hypothyroidism and bone density issues occur at the same time, it's because the virus is behind both. (To counteract the calcium loss, you'll find the surprising best food sources of calcium in Chapter 22, "Powerful Foods, Herbs, and Supplements for Healing.")

Metabolism Problems

The concept of metabolism as the driving force of weight gain, weight loss, and hunger is a myth. It's a very broad and outdated term that distracts from the truth that so much is still unknown in medical communities about why people suffer in this area. If you've been told you have a faulty metabolism, don't let it derail you. You don't have a faulty metabolism, and *you're* not faulty, either. There's a real cause that's behind your struggles, and it's one that you can address with this book. To help you pinpoint the true source of your issue, see the explanations of the next few symptoms.

Mystery Weight Gain

Mysterious weight gain is a common symptom that leaves many people beyond frustrated. You're watching what you eat, you're exercising regularly, and the number on the scale keeps going up. You might have heard that this is a result of a hypothyroid—that you have an underactive thyroid that's failing to produce enough metabolism-boosting hormones to keep your weight in check. This isn't how it works. As you'll read about in "Great Mistake 5: The Metabolism Myth," *metabolism* is one of those broad-sweeping terms that covers up the fact that not much is known about the true mechanics of weight gain. If underproduction of thyroid hormones were the true explanation for it, then how to explain all the people with hypothyroidism who don't experience this symptom?

Here's what's really going on: Back when the Epstein-Barr virus was in Stage Two and hiding out in your liver, it weakened the organ and burdened it to the point of creating a sluggish liver. Then, even after the virus moved on to the thyroid, some EBV cells remained in the liver, where they could continue to cause trouble as they fed and prospered on antibiotics, other old pharmaceuticals, pesticides, herbicides, toxic heavy metals, solvents, and more in that organ. Plus, EBV's presence in the body results in the ongoing presence of viral byproduct, dead virus cells, neurotoxins, and dermatoxins

in the system that give the liver and lymphatic system continuous purifying work to do, so they keep getting strained. All of that and the adrenal glands that are overcompensating for the underactive thyroid flood the liver with excess adrenaline, giving it even more of a toxic load. Essentially, the liver becomes spiced with the toxins, pickled with adrenaline, and can't do its job properly anymore, then foists off whatever it can to the lymphatic system. (You don't need to have adrenal fatigue to have a liver that's saturated with adrenaline.)

It's the resulting overburdened, sluggish liver and lymphatic system that are behind a hypothyroid patient's tendency to have difficulty losing weight or to gain pounds without control. So *both* the hypothyroid and the weight gain are caused by the virus. It's *not* the hypothyroid itself causing the weight gain.

It's also not unusual for someone with a hyperthyroid to experience weight gain. In truth, more people with a hyperthyroid struggle with weight gain than loss. This fact that most hyperthyroid patients are overweight baffles medical communities—it's a fact that's not taken seriously and therefore ignored because it goes against the "rules" carved out for what defines hyperthyroidism. However, in reality, it makes plenty of sense. The types of EBV that cause hyperthyroidism are just as disruptive to the liver as those varieties that cause hypothyroidism. Eventually, a hyperthyroid patient's liver gets clogged and overburdened, too, and the result is trouble keeping off the pounds.

Much of mysterious extra weight gain is fluid retention. For instance, if you think you're 60 pounds overweight, it's probably only 40 pounds of body fat, and the other 20 pounds are fluid that your body's holding on to—a proportion that medical communities don't yet realize. Why does this fluid retention happen?

Because when the liver gets to the point where it can't protect you from toxins in the bloodstream anymore, your lymphatic system must step in to become the filter your liver's meant to be. Your lymphatic system is geared to be an after-filter to the liver, dealing with micro and nano amounts of toxins and debris. However, when the liver gets pre-fatty, fatty, sluggish, stagnant, or even just sick—conditions that can slip by a doctor—and can't do its job anymore, the lymphatic system must take on all the macro waste matter that the liver can't handle. Since this sludge is thicker than the lymphatic system is meant to handle, it clogs the lymphatic vessels and lymph ducts, so lymph fluid can't flow as it normally would. To adapt to this, the lymphatic system tries to push lymph fluid around it with the goal of building pressure to flush out the large-scale debris; however the lymph generally still can't flow through the passageways unhampered, so pockets of fluid start to collect. The result is that you retain fluid, adding inches to your waistline and pounds to the scale as a case of underlying, undiagnosed lymphedema develops.

It's worth noting that even if you haven't been diagnosed with a thyroid condition, a viral infection of the thyroid and the effects I just described could still be behind your struggles to lose weight. As I mentioned earlier and as we'll look at in more detail in Chapter 7, thyroid testing isn't yet what it could be, so a thyroid panel won't necessarily show if your hormone levels are low.

Many alternative-minded M.D.s, including functional or integrative doctors, are examining the thyroid now more than ever because they think it's the explanation behind mysterious weight gain. They're thoroughly examining blood-test results, and even when the tests don't show any signs of thyroid troubles, they're offering thyroid medication for certain patients based on all the other evidence with their health. This is a step forward in that patients are getting well-deserved attention and not just told they're overweight because they're lazy or that stepping on the treadmill will solve their problems. And yet thyroid medication to solve weight gain is still not an answer—because it's not an underactive thyroid that's the problem to begin with.

If you're on medication for a thyroid condition and you're still struggling with your weight and wondering why, it's because the medicine isn't healing the underlying viral infection, thyroid damage, or liver issue. Further, thyroid medications are hard on the liver and the adrenals; they make the adrenals work overtime, which saturates the liver, and the liver is already working at trying to process the medication itself. This slows down the liver additionally, meaning that someone's weight can increase even more over time when on thyroid medication, or that medication can trigger weight gain if it wasn't a problem in the first place. (More on thyroid medication in Chapter 8.)

The reason that some people experience weight loss when they begin thyroid prescriptions is that they overhauled their diet and started new exercise and supplementation regimens at the same time (a combination that's very helpful for bringing back a tired liver) while also often cutting out some of the foods that feed EBV. (There's an exceedingly small group of people who experience weight loss on thyroid medication without taking any other measures. This is due to the initial shock of the body receiving a foreign steroid hormone compound. Ultimately, these individuals will gain weight again, because the viral issue is not addressed.) If you don't address the underlying viral and liver issues with the techniques in this book, the weight gain continues—and women usually end up hearing it's a result of menopause, which isn't the truth at all. (For the full story on menopause, see the chapter "Premenstrual Syndrome and Menopause" in *Medical Medium*.)

Mystery Weight Loss

The mysterious weight loss that some people with thyroid issues experience is not due to a hyperthyroid. There are thousands of people with hyperthyroidism, and they are gaining weight or overweight. That's right—while you may have a thyroid that's overproducing thyroid hormones, it's not those hormones making it difficult to keep or put on weight. Once again, this is a viral symptom. Certain varieties of EBV release poisons that are allergenic to the body, which prompts a constant flow of adrenaline—and for some people, that translates to weight loss, because the hormone basically acts like an amphetamine. (It's also very common to have difficulty sleeping alongside this rapid weight loss, due to the excess adrenaline in the system.) Most people with weight loss issues eventually experience the opposite, either a year or ten years down the road, as adrenal fatigue sets in and their symptom flips to weight gain instead.

Constant Hunger

Though this symptom is commonly associated with a hyperthyroid, most people with a hypothyroid also experience periods of nagging, constant, or almost insatiable hunger, too. That's because this symptom isn't tied to the thyroid; it's due to glycogen (stored glucose) deficiencies in the liver and/or brain—and EBV

is to blame. When EBV spends a long time in the liver, it requires a lot of energy from the organ, which means the liver burns through fuel and can easily become deficient in glycogen. The virus also causes central nervous system weaknesses, and since the central nervous system requires sugar to function, too, it goes through glucose at a rapid rate—and wants more fast. The result of a brain and/or liver glycogen deficiency is a feeling of hunger as your body cries out for more of it. (Note that a high-fat/low-carb diet only makes the situation worse, as healthy carbohydrates contain the sugars you need, and too much fat in the diet both hinders the body's conversion and absorption of these natural sugars and also weakens the liver.)

Mystery Hair Thinning and Hair Loss

Mysterious hair thinning and hair loss are also symptomatic of EBV's damaging presence. It's not low production of thyroid hormones that causes clumps of hair to fall out in your hand—it's excess adrenaline and cortisol. The adrenal glands are the most important glands in the endocrine system. They are the mediators of the body. So as we saw, when the thyroid is struggling, the adrenals jump in to produce extra hormones. Once in a while, this would be fine. When the thyroid is constantly struggling due to viral infection, though, and the adrenals are constantly filling in for them, the repeated floods of stress chemicals are hard on the body and can cause hair to thin and/or fall out.

These changes in your hair aren't always immediate. Because it takes some time to see the effects of stress-hormone-saturated hair follicles, it could be six to nine months, or even a year, after EBV has reached the thyroid before you start seeing differences in your hair.

If you have no other symptoms, it could be that you don't have the thyroid virus at all, and your mystery hair thinning or loss is due to an experience from months ago that caused surges of stress chemicals at the time. Break-ups, other relationship upheavals, and child-birth are all common examples of when you might find yourself shedding months later. You may be perfectly content by then, with every-thing blown over, and suddenly your shower drain starts filling with hair. That's because of that same lag time it takes for the hair follicles to weaken.

On the other hand, if you're constantly overstressed or have nutritional deficiencies, that timeline for hair thinning or loss (whether viral-caused, stress-related, or both) can be much shorter. People who are prone to eczema (more on this skin affliction soon) tend to experience greater hair loss due to their already irritated scalps.

Another common reason for hair loss is the use of thyroid medications, antibiotics, or other pharmaceuticals. I've seen hundreds upon hundreds of cases where women start to lose hair shortly after going on thyroid medications—even though they were given those medications in part because of hair thinning that was thought to be from a thyroid condition.

Sometimes it seems as though thyroid medication stops hair loss at first. This is only because of coincidental timing. As I said, it's not uncommon for a woman to go through a stressful period in her life that results in hair loss months later, seemingly out of the blue. Her doctor will suspect thyroid trouble, put her on thyroid hormones, and lo and behold, she'll stop losing hair. In reality, it wasn't the effect of the medication. The patient stopped shedding only because her adrenals had started to recover from the stress by that time, giving her hair follicles a break so they could recover, too. The hair loss would have stopped without the medication; the medication had masked the ability to benchmark the body's natural healing process. If the patient continues on the prescription, there's a good chance that a few months later, her hair will begin to fall out again, confusing both patient and doctor, because they thought the medication was the fix.

And in some cases, radiation exposure can cause hair thinning. One dental X-ray can be enough to thin hair for about a month or two.

Change in Hair Texture

A change in hair texture that makes it brittle or coarser than usual is commonly due to EBV inside the liver giving off internal dermatoxins that reach the scalp, combined with years of nutritional deficiencies and adrenal surges. Another reason hair can lose luster is because as your body fights EBV, it directs the nutritional resources such as trace minerals, vitamins, and antioxidants that would normally go toward keeping your hair healthy toward supporting your body against the virus instead.

Insomnia

As with the other symptoms you'll find in this list, insomnia is not a symptom of thyroid trouble. Even though you'll read in the latest literature about this thyroid-insomnia trend, the truth is that a compromised thyroid does not disrupt sleep. Insomnia may *accompany* thyroid issues, if the virus is disrupting both this endocrine gland and your neurotransmitters at the same time, which is common. Or your troubled sleep could be attributable to any number of other hidden causes of insomnia and sleep disturbances, including emotional wounds, digestive sensitivities, liver issues, obsessive-compulsive disorder (OCD), worry, and MSG toxicity. The entire last section of this book, Part IV, "Secrets of Sleep," is devoted to helping you figure out the reason for your individual case of troubled sleep so you can start using sleep to heal—in part by learning about the unknown laws of sleep.

Fatigue

This common symptom can occur at different stages of EBV. Early on, during the mono phase, fatigue can result as your immune system puts its energy into fighting your first active, present, and ready-to-go-into-action viral blood infection.

Once EBV is in the organs, a second type of fatigue—neurological fatigue—can occur from the virus releasing its neurotoxins. Neurological fatigue is frequently mistaken for adrenal fatigue, though they are truly distinct. Neurological fatigue and adrenal fatigue can occur either separately or at the same time, because one has to do with the nervous system and the other with the endocrine system.

Adrenal fatigue is a real and legitimate condition—there's a reason that I devoted a chapter to it in *Medical Medium*. Still, we must be careful not to identify every case of fatigue as adrenal fatigue—which is what's happening in many medical communities today. Doctors, other practitioners, and the latest books are pointing to adrenal overload as the explanation for so much. It's not the brand-new discovery it may seem like. It's recycled and repackaged information that's technically decades old in its attempt to explain why so many people are sidelined in life. Adrenal fatigue as the across-the-board answer is distracting from the truth, which is that late-stage Epstein-Barr virus is targeting the central nervous systems of countless people. Viral neurotoxins are flooding their systems, creating an undetectable viral encephalitis (brain inflammation) that creates irritated, lethargic, sensitive nerves throughout the body and can get in the way of life in devastating ways.

The practical difference between these two types of fatigue is that with adrenal fatigue, people can still function. They can work, hold down jobs, socialize, exercise, and care for family, though they don't feel terribly vital while doing any of it. Neurological fatigue, on the other hand, has a flatline effect. The fatigue is so pronounced that your ability to function in normal society gets taken away. While severe adrenal fatigue does happen, and adrenal fatigue and neurological fatigue can also occur at the same time (which is when people struggle the most), neurological fatigue on its own is the common type that accompanies advanced EBV.

With a mild case of neurological fatigue, you may get extremely tired from driving your car a short distance, feel like your legs are a ton of bricks, experience weakness in your arms in various ways, battle heavy confusion, and have difficulty finding the strength to bathe or make a meal. With a more advanced case of neurological fatigue, when neurotoxins flood and saturate the brain, you may feel like you couldn't get yourself out of bed even if your life depended on it. Severe neurological fatigue like this is what has the roughly 17 out of 100 college students I mentioned earlier dropping out of school and spiraling into despair.

Tiredness

A feeling of tiredness that overwork and stress don't explain, and that you can't shake despite getting enough sleep, is a milder form of fatigue that EBV can cause. In this case, it's the low-grade viral infection straining your immune system and organs while draining your energy levels.

Changes in Energy Levels

Sometimes fatigue, exhaustion, and tiredness come and go. On a regular basis, this can either be a sign that you're at the beginning of a very low-grade viral infection that hasn't had time to settle in yet, or it means you can detox fairly well. On a bad day, you've filled up with the EBV neurotoxins and other viral waste, and they're making it difficult to function. On a good day, your body has cleansed the toxic matter, and you're free to live your life. Most of the time, this accompanies underactive or overactive adrenals due to stresses or triggers in your life that have instigated adrenal instability. This usually prompts the doctor to overlook everything else that's wrong and diagnose you with adrenal fatigue or cortisol issues as the main problem. If you were worse off, with a stagnant liver and a toxic digestive tract, you wouldn't experience much fluctuation in energy levels; your energy would stay consistently low.

Brain Fog and Difficulty Concentrating

A fuzzy or foggy mental feeling that keeps you from being able to think clearly happens when EBV is feeding off of its favorite foods, which include toxic heavy metals such as mercury, as well as dairy products, eggs, wheat, corn, excess adrenaline, and prescription drugs. As EBV feasts and prospers, it gives off more waste, and these neurotoxins travel to the brain and short-circuit neurotransmitters. When focus issues define your brain fog, it's usually due to an extra abundance of heavy metals in the brain coupled with that short-circuiting. This can often lead to a mistaken diagnosis of attention-deficit/hyperactivity disorder (ADHD), leaky gut, parasitical infection, Lyme disease, or a thyroid disorder.

Memory Loss

Memory issues happen for the same basic reason as brain fog, with EBV devouring its favorite foods in your system and loading you down with that much more disruptive waste. In this case, someone has higher elevations of mercury and other toxic heavy metals, both of which give the virus extra fuel, which translates to extra neurotoxic waste matter short-circuiting neurotransmitter activity. Additionally, when those heavy metals oxidize in the brain or liver, the toxic runoff saturates brain tissue, smothering electrical impulses—and getting in the way of proper memory function.

Heightened Sensitivity to Cold

A tendency to "run cold" and need to wear extra layers to stay warm happens because of high elevations of viral neurotoxins in your system that make your nerves sensitive to colder temperatures. This is often mistaken for a metabolism issue when it's really a sensitive nerve issue.

Cold Hands and Feet

When you often find that your extremities are cold, it's the viral neurotoxins causing nerve sensitivity to low temperatures, *plus* a sluggish liver causing a circulation issue.

Chills

Frequent chills and shivers on a chronic level that aren't related to cold, flu, overheating, or dehydration are signs that your immune system is fighting an EBV infection in the organs too deep in the body for doctors to detect with a blood test.

Hot Flashes and Night Sweats

Bursts of feeling hot and sweaty out of nowhere are caused by a toxic liver—not by the thyroid *or* menopause. Hot flashes and night sweats have nothing to do with hormones. Here's what's really going on: When the liver fills up with toxins such as viral poisons, heavy metals, pesticides, herbicides, and even old storage of prescription drugs, it becomes overburdened and starts to run hot—so the body tries to cool it down. As part of this process, heat is expelled from the liver and pulsed through the body, giving you that uncomfortable overheated sensation. This is a very common experience for both women and men, though because of the stigma, men's hot flashes aren't normally labeled as such. They're often called "work sweats" or "nervous sweats" instead.

Running Hot

A tendency to feel overheated is another sign of liver heat and the body's work to release it. You may go back and forth between running hot and running cold—this is not at all unusual and has to do with the body fighting to cool itself and drawing energy from the spleen.

Excessive Sweating

When a low-grade viral load of EBV releases neurotoxins that contain large amounts of mercury, it creates a strained and sensitive central nervous system. Those mercury-filled neurotoxins short-circuit neurotransmitters and block electrical impulses, which sends mixed messages throughout the brain. The result is a sensation of nervousness. Even if someone doesn't feel emotionally nervous, the body gets the message to go into an anxious response, and this prompts the production of extra sweat.

Body Temperature Fluctuations

If your doctor or practitioner has diagnosed you with a thyroid condition due to body temperature fluctuations, and if you don't have adrenal issues, hypoglycemia, or insulin resistance—then in its mild form, this is one of those rare symptoms that can be related to the thyroid (as a result of low thyroid hormones or excess thyroid hormones). More noticeable chills and hot flashes are generally caused by EBV, as explained above.

Edema

Unless you have a true heart condition or kidney disease that's on your doctor's radar, this swelling happens as a result of EBV and its sludge in the bloodstream and lymphatic system. As with mystery weight gain, a liver that's filled with viral sewage from EBV becomes sluggish or even stagnant, handing off its filtration duties to the lymphatic system, which in turn retains pockets of fluid because it's not equipped to process this large-scale waste matter.

Puffy Face and/or Puffy Eyes

One common reason for this symptom is a form of lymphedema where fluid is retained in the face and eye area for the same reason as above. You'll usually find that the puffiness comes and goes. That's because the body's elevations of toxins go up and down as new ones come in and some old ones are processed out through urine and other avenues of detoxification.

Puffiness can also occur due to viral-related allergic reaction. If your diet contains foods that feed EBV (see Chapter 21, "Common Misconceptions and What to Avoid"), you can develop an allergy to the toxic byproduct that the virus eliminates after fueling itself on those foods. Because this byproduct is an even more allergenic, Frankensteined version of the food, you could be allergic to this waste even if you don't react to the food itself. It drives up homocysteine and inflammation levels (and may make any allergy tests you get go haywire), resulting in that puffiness. Again, this is not a thyroid-caused symptom.

Swollen Hands and Feet

Swelling of your hands and feet happens for two reasons: (1) a histamine variety of edema, in which the body is reacting to EBV's neurotoxins with elevated histamines that flood the lymphatic system and the bloodstream, and/or (2) liver and lymphatic sluggishness due to being overburdened with viral waste matter and other toxins, such as heavy metals. It's very common for someone in this situation to receive a diagnosis of idiopathic (unknown cause) lupus or even Lyme disease.

Mood Swings

When EBV feeds off of its favorite foods such as wheat gluten, dairy products, eggs, and heavy metals in your system, it excretes neurotoxins that fill the bloodstream, interfere with your neurotransmitters, and make you feel less vital. As a result, your mood can drop until the virus's feeding frenzy has died down and your vitality has returned.

These mood swings can tax the adrenals, which puts strain on your liver and pancreas. Plus this viral waste matter in the bloodstream can even tamper with your blood sugar levels to the point of hypoglycemia, which further contributes to mood ups and downs, creating a vicious cycle until you crack the EBV code and discover how to stop feeding the virus. This hypoglycemia may be a mild version that flies under the radar of diagnostics. It's also possible for these mood issues to result in a mistaken diagnosis of bipolar disorder.

Irritability

In women, this symptom is almost always blamed on a hormone issue. Here's what's really going on: When EBV neurotoxins short out neurotransmitters in the brain, it typically leads to irritability, crankiness, and even unexplained anger or sadness, which for most women leads to a depression diagnosis at the doctor's office. When this neurotoxin activity is accompanied by a toxic, sluggish liver, irritability can amplify. And if you have particularly large deposits of heavy metals such as mercury in the brain, this symptom can be severe.

Anxiety

Far too many people are told that their anxiety is behind their health problems—that if they could learn to control their worries, they'd be in much better shape. In reality, it's the other way around: Physical health issues are behind almost the entire anxiety epidemic. When anxiety is not stand-alone and accompanies other symptoms in this list, at least part of that physical cause is usually a large amount of EBV neurotoxins that are saturating and inflaming the vagus nerve (which runs to the brain), along with elevated levels of toxic heavy metals.

While emotional trauma can also cause anxiety all on its own, that anxiety so often sticks around, even when the trauma is long past, and becomes chronic because of a vicious cycle with EBV: anxious periods trigger off bursts of fear-based adrenaline, which fuels the virus, in turn releasing an abundance of neurotoxins that keep anxiety going. For more on anxiety, turn to Chapter 29, "Identifying Sleep Issues."

Depression

Like anxiety, depression is frequently blamed as the origin of someone's physical suffering, when the truth is that depression can be traced to physical origins. Depression is not the sign of a weak mind or character; it's a very real symptom that can give you important insights into your health. If depression accompanies other symptoms on this list, EBV is a likely culprit. When EBV feeds off of large amounts of toxic heavy metals in your system, the resulting high levels of neurotoxic waste saturate the brain, altering and hampering neurotransmitters such as dopamine and serotonin—resulting in a depressive state. This means that depression is not something anyone can "snap out of" or wish away—though you can certainly find relief from it by detoxing the virus along with its food (including heavy metals) and waste. For more on depression, see the chapter devoted to it in *Medical Medium*.

Restlessness

The feeling that you can't quite settle down or relax is often due, once again, to EBV neurotoxins. If these poisons are in your organs, they can create an allergic sensation that translates to physical unease such as anxiousness, restlessness, and a can't-sit-still kind of feeling.

Restless Legs

Often diagnosed as idiopathic, mysterious anxiety, restless legs syndrome is in fact due to high levels of toxic heavy metals and an elevated viral load in the brain or other areas of the nervous system. This neurological symptom that often interferes with sleep occurs when these heavy metals and EBV's neurotoxins interfere with neurotransmitters and neurons, causing electrical impulses to take paths they're not meant to, effectively short-circuiting. The resulting messages gone awry can create that uncomfortable leg sensation—or it can even cause restless arms or a restless torso.

Aches and Pains

It's extremely common for EBV's neurotoxins to create achy feelings throughout the body. When combined with EBV's dermatoxins, the result can be psoriatic arthritis—joint pain from the neurotoxins with psoriasis on the skin from the dermatoxins.

Headaches and Migraines

When EBV produces neurotoxins, they often travel up to the brain, where they interfere with electrical impulses, which can cause headaches. If you have a really high viral load of EBV plus toxic heavy metals in your system, then migraines can be triggered as a result of EBV flaring up the phrenic and/or vagus nerves. When you also have the shingles virus (it's possible to have both shingles and the thyroid virus), it can cause inflammation of the trigeminal nerve, which can trigger a migraine that affects the ear, jaw, face, or side of the head. (For a more thorough look at migraines, see the chapter about them in *Medical Medium*.)

Joint Pain

Often, late-stage EBV specifically attacks joints, cartilage, and/or connective tissue, inflaming the nerves in those areas in the process. The result is stiff, painful, swollen, or even misshapen joints (as in rheumatoid arthritis).

Muscle Cramps

A liver that's grown sluggish and fatty due to EBV and other factors such as pesticides, antibiotics, other pharmaceuticals, toxic chemicals, unproductive food, and toxic heavy metals can contribute to magnesium, potassium, glucose, and glycogen deficiencies, because the liver is meant to be their storage bin, and when it grows weak, it loses its ability to hold on to them. These nutrients all feed muscles, so deficiencies can translate to cramped muscles.

Muscle Weakness

Muscle weakness is a part of the neurological fatigue I mentioned earlier in this chapter. When EBV's neurotoxins get to the brain, they can cause very mild, undetectable encephalitis (brain inflammation) that affects the nervous system and weakens muscles. In many cases, it will be misdiagnosed as MS or Lyme disease at the doctor's office. When someone has both adrenal fatigue and neurological fatigue at the same time, this weakness can be worse. However, this symptom can occur as a result of neurological fatigue alone, too.

Tingles and Numbness

When EBV's neurotoxins inflame nerves, tingles and numbness can result. If this symptom occurs in the tongue or face, the vagus nerve is inflamed. If it's in the hands or arms, the phrenic nerves, which run through the chest, are inflamed. If the tingling and/or numbness occurs in the legs and feet, the neurotoxins are inflaming the pudendal nerve, tibial nerve, and/or sciatic nerve. Though often mistaken for neuropathy or even transient ischemic attack (TIA), this symptom rarely equates to permanent nerve damage.

Twitches and Spasms

When EBV feeds off of mercury and as a result releases neurotoxins high in methylmercury byproduct, those neurotoxins are prone to short-circuiting neurotransmitters in the brain—which reduces neuron strength and interferes with electrical impulses in the brain. These neurotoxins also lower magnesium, sodium, glucose, glycogen, and B_{12} levels to the point of severe nervous system deficiencies that are not yet detectable through blood testing.

Trembling Hands

EBV's neurotoxins absorb and diffuse neurotransmitters, which can ultimately lead to neurotransmitter deficiency, in turn causing these tremors. A higher level of toxic heavy metals is often present with this symptom, which is sometimes misdiagnosed as a sign of Parkinson's. Neurotransmitter deficiency can also arise as a result of EBV's neurotoxins, mostly mercury-based ones, triggering overactive adrenals—because excess adrenaline can burn out neurotransmitters.

Heart Palpitations, Ectopic Heartbeats, Arrhythmia

So often, mystery heart palpitations, skipped beats, and irregular heartbeats do not originate with the heart. Instead, we need to look to the Epstein-Barr virus and its effects on the liver. That's right: EBV's byproduct and viral corpses form a sticky, jelly-like sludge that builds up in the liver—until the organ gets oversaturated, at which point the substance begins to break apart and get sucked into the heart. The result is that heart valves, particularly the mitral valve, can get gummed up with the buildup and start to stick instead of allowing for the free flow of blood.

Heart palpitations can also occur as a result of Stage Four EBV producing a tremendous amount of neurotoxins that affect the brain and vagus nerve, translating to neurologically caused heart-rate irregularities.

In neither of these cases are the heart flutters life-threatening or related to the thyroid—they are, instead, an EBV-caused nuisance.

Changes in Heart Rate

When the central nervous system becomes hypersensitive due to the onslaught of neurotoxins in late-stage EBV, the brain's messaging to the adrenal glands becomes extremely inconsistent. Consequently, the adrenals get various messages either to produce at full force or slow to a crawl, and your heart rate speeds up or slows accordingly, because adrenaline is linked to heart rate. Since it's not outside stimulus such as stress or relaxation that's causing your adrenals to pump harder or back off, the effect on your heart rate can feel random and unprompted. It's very common for these changes in heart rate to accompany other adrenal-related conditions, including Cushing's syndrome, Addison's disease (both of these are caused by EBV), and posttraumatic stress disorder (PTSD).

Tightness in the Chest

A sensation of tightness in the chest can be caused by EBV and/or its neurotoxins inflaming the vagus and phrenic nerves, sometimes resulting in unexplained anxiety or a panic diagnosis.

Hypertension (High Blood Pressure)

If you've been diagnosed with hypertension and doctors haven't been able to identify a cardiovascular issue that's causing it, there's a good chance a sluggish or stagnant liver is the explanation. That's because the heart draws clean blood from the liver, an arrangement that works smoothly if the liver—the body's filter—is in good condition. When the liver is compromised, though—whether stiffened from scar tissue (caused by EBV's damage to the organ), clogged with a high-fat diet, overloaded with EBV waste matter and other toxins, or all of the above—it can't filter as well, so instead of passing along toxic debris to the kidneys and intestinal tract for elimination, sludge builds up and backs up into the bloodstream and lymphatic system. This means that blood becomes "dirtier" and thicker, which makes the heart work harder to pull it up.

To picture this, think of a glass of water. How easy is it to suck that water up through a straw? Pretty easy. How about a can of cola? Since it's a little syrupy, you'll have to work a little harder to bring the liquid up. Now what

about a milkshake? That liquid is much thicker, so you need to create that much more suction to draw it up the straw. That's how it works with the heart trying to draw up thick blood—it requires more pressure.

High Cholesterol

A liver that's sluggish, filled with toxins, pre-fatty, or fatty due to a high-protein/high-fat diet and EBV's toxic load is a common reason for a high cholesterol reading.

Tinnitus (Ringing or Buzzing in the Ears)

In Stage Four, EBV can target the nerves of the inner ear labyrinth, and the resulting inflammation and vibration can lead to ringing or buzzing sensations, or even unexplained deafening. That's the most common explanation for tinnitus.

Alternately, EBV's neurotoxins can inflame those nerves of the inner ear, and the mere exposure of these nerves to the neurotoxins can create this symptom.

Vertigo, Ménière's Disease, Dizziness, Balance Issues

This symptom is not a result of calcium crystals or stones becoming disrupted in the inner ear. Rather, when EBV is leaving the thyroid as it moves into Stage Four, it's usually moving fast, growing rapidly in number—and will often release an explosion of neurotoxins into the bloodstream. The vagus and even phrenic nerves become sensitized and allergic to the neurotoxins, causing them to inflame, which causes "the spins" and other disconcerting balance issues. When the vagus nerve swells like this, it causes the chest and neck to get tight, and, since the nerve runs into the cranium, it even results in some very mild inflammation at the bottom of the brain. This swelling of the brain itself (which is on such a minute scale it can't be detected with MRIs or CT scans) can compound the balance issues, going so far as to give you a chronic balance issue where you feel like you're constantly on a boat, or aboard a flight that's always in a turbulent landing phase.

Goiter

The goiter of today is an infection of EBV in the thyroid that causes fluid buildup and swelling. Very rarely is a goiter caused by a simple case of iodine deficiency, as in yesteryear.

Throat Tightness

This is often another symptom of EBV creating vagus nerve inflammation. Since the vagus nerve runs through the throat area, when EBV's neurotoxins inflame it, or when virus cells grab on to exposed root hairs of the nerve, it can create an uncomfortable sensation of tightness.

In some cases, throat tightness is caused by a thyroid that's become especially inflamed and enlarged by EBV.

Swollen Tongue

Vagus nerve inflammation can create a chain of nerve inflammation—which means that nerves in the tongue can become inflamed from EBV, too, resulting in swelling of the organ.

Altered Sense of Taste and Smell

Again, an inflamed vagus nerve, caused by EBV neurotoxins or virus cells, can cause inflammation in the nerves that branch off from it. This can affect the tongue and taste buds and/or the nasal cavity.

Metallic Taste in the Mouth

When EBV feeds off of high levels of toxic heavy metals such as mercury in your system and the virus's neurotoxins in your bloodstream consequently contain high levels of heavy metals, you can end up with a metallic taste in your mouth. You can also get a metallic taste when you're actively detoxing heavy metals and they aren't being passed along by a full "team" of heavy metal–eliminating foods and supplements. (For more on heavy metal detoxification, see Chapter 23, "90-Day Thyroid Rehab.")

Hoarseness or Change in Voice

Mild inflammation of the thyroid from EBV is enough to create this symptom. Another common cause is EBV-related chronic acid reflux (more on this soon). Lastly, dairy, eggs, and wheat are highly mucus-forming foods and fuel for EBV; eating them prompts the virus to produce extra waste matter that overloads the lymphatic system and can result in a hoarse voice.

Brittle or Ridged Nails

Zinc is one of the most important resources to fight EBV. The body uses up supplies and even deep reserves of zinc at a rapid rate—meaning that it's very common to become zinc-deficient when you have EBV, if you weren't already. This zinc deficiency is responsible for issues with your nails.

Dry, Cracking Skin

When the liver can't function properly anymore as a result of EBV infection, it often gets to the point where it can't handle fats—it can't process them or protect the bloodstream from too much of them. Higher elevations of fat in the bloodstream reduce oxygen levels delivered to the dermis; less oxygen means that the toxins can't be flushed out of the skin properly. This means that the skin ends up harboring toxins, which cause the skin to become inflamed and even to erupt in cracks as it tries to release those poisons.

Constipation

The most common cause of chronic constipation is a sluggish, fatty, or stagnant liver overburdened from a high-fat diet and overloaded from the presence of EBV and heavy metals. At the same time, EBV's cofactor bacteria, strep, often proliferates in the digestive tract, causing inflammation in various parts of the gut.

Constipation can also occur as a result of EBV's neurotoxins floating up to the brain through the bloodstream, weakening the central nervous system and creating neurological fatigue, which slows down signals from the brain to the colon for peristaltic action.

Chronic Diarrhea

A sick, sluggish, stagnant, fatty, or scarred liver, along with an inflamed pancreas and high levels of EBV's cofactor, strep bacteria, inside the gut can—when they occur on a chronic, long-term basis—trigger the body's elimination response. Further, when the liver releases large amounts of EBV byproduct and other sludge into the intestines, the intestinal lining can become agitated and inflamed and try to eliminate it quickly through diarrhea. Also, both EBV and strep feed off of foods such as milk, cheese, butter, eggs, corn, canola, and GMO soy, so these foods in the diet result in more intestinal agitation, allowing for conditions such as irritable bowel syndrome (IBS), Crohn's, and celiac.

Loss of Libido

Yet again, this is a symptom that is not thyroid-caused. Plenty of people with hypothyroidism and Hashimoto's have plenty of libido. In truth, women's sex drive is determined by their adrenal strength. This is a protective mechanism of the body; if the adrenals don't have enough reserves for giving birth, then it triggers a shutoff switch for libido. (Men, on the other hand, can have compromised adrenals and plenty of libido.)

Abnormal Menstrual Periods

Inconsistent menstrual flows and cycles can occur for a few different reasons, none of them thyroid-related. The first common reason is due to a chronic infection of EBV in the uterus and ovaries. Remember, in the second phase of Stage Two EBV, the virus can enter the reproductive organs. Whether it's to the point of causing uterine fibroids or ovarian cysts yet or not, the virus's presence can disrupt the normal function of the reproductive system.

Adrenal dysfunction caused by EBV is another possible explanation if you experience inconsistent menstrual cycles. Also, a diet too high in protein, fat, dairy, and eggs can cause menstruation issues.

Blurry Vision and Other Vision Problems

When you experience mysterious blurry vision that a visit to the optometrist, ophthalmologist, and/or a prescription for eyeglasses can't explain or correct, it's likely due to EBV neurotoxins in the bloodstream that are (1) short-circuiting and diminishing neurotransmitters, and (2) weakening the optic nerve.

Epstein-Barr virus cells can also get into the eye itself and cause destruction there, sometimes going so far as to cause a detached retina or glaucoma. The shingles virus has the ability to weaken optic nerves as well.

Eye Floaters

EBV neurotoxins inflaming the optic nerve can create mirage-like experiences of black spots, white spots, glares, and white flashes in the eyes.

Bulging Eyes

This symptom is commonly associated with Graves' disease and hyperthyroidism, though it should be noted that it doesn't occur with every case of these—and that it's not your body itself creating the problem. Once again, the underlying cause here is EBV: When certain aggressive varieties of the virus prompt the thyroid gland to produce more tissue, that extra tissue produces extra thyroid hormones—and these excess steroid compounds create the swelling that causes eyes to bulge. It's a steroid response; the same would happen to someone continuously taking a large amount of human growth hormone.

Skin Discoloration

When you're dealing with a low-grade EBV infection that's causing the liver to be dysfunctional, it can create bilirubin problems that don't show up on blood tests as full-on jaundice. Instead, your thyroid may be blamed if you present with just a bit of extra yellow pigmentation in your skin. Make no mistake: This symptom has nothing to do with a hypothyroid. It's a liver issue.

As you've found repeatedly in this symptom list, the liver plays a huge role in your health. When someone has had EBV percolating in her or his liver for a long time, and especially when that person has also taken a decent amount of antibiotics or other medications in her or his day, the liver can become too overburdened to process bilirubin, the yellow pigment formed by the breakdown of old blood cells, correctly. Instead of getting flushed out, the bilirubin builds up and backs up into the bloodstream, resulting in that yellowish tinge to the skin.

For an explanation of circulation-related skin discoloration, see "Raynaud's Syndrome" in the next section.

WHAT YOUR OTHER HEALTH PROBLEMS MEAN

People who struggle with thyroid disorders often struggle with additional health issues that are mistaken for separate problems. It can feel very disheartening to walk around with multiple diagnoses—not only may you feel as though there's something wrong with you as a person that you can't just be healthier; you may also walk around waiting for the other shoe to drop, concerned that if you have an autoimmune thyroid diagnosis, then that makes you predisposed to develop more autoimmune diseases along the way.

Don't let these worries burden your heart any longer. The reality is that EBV is behind so many health issues—many of them autoimmune—that there's an extremely likely chance that it's not many separate, unrelated symptoms and conditions you're dealing with or fearing. Rather, they may all come from the same source. All conditions caused by EBV, including chronic fatigue syndrome, rheumatoid arthritis, Lyme disease, fibromyalgia, and lupus, tend to coexist alongside thyroid issues, because it's the same virus causing them all. Since you're discovering how to free yourself from the virus with this book, you'll have the tools you need to address the true root of your problem and finally move on with your life.

Let's look at some of the most common conditions that people experience alongside thyroid issues. Remember, these aren't the standard answers you'll find from other resources.

Perimenopause and Menopause

Hot flashes, weight gain, hair loss, memory loss, fatigue, brain fog—there's a tremendous amount of confusion out there about whether to attribute these to thyroid disease or menopause. A woman may receive a "change of life" diagnosis alongside or instead of a thyroid diagnosis, either way giving her the sense that her body is rebelling and aging her rapidly.

The truth is that these symptoms are due to neither thyroid dysfunction nor hormonal transition nor aging. Much of the time, EBV is the cause—in the previous part of the chapter, you read about how the virus is capable of creating all of these symptoms. It's also possible for radiation or pesticide exposure to contribute to the discomforts classically associated with menopause.

As I described in detail in the first book of the Medical Medium series, menopause is not meant to be a painful, uncomfortable process, and in fact marks the beginning of slowed-down aging. It just so happened that historically, the incubation period for EBV was such that it started to infect the thyroid and cause symptoms at the same time a woman's menstrual periods were stopping, and the coincidence was mistaken for causation. These days, with more aggressive, faster-developing strains of EBV showcasing themselves, women are coming down with hypothyroidism earlier in life, and now it's not uncommon for 25-year-olds or even college students to receive diagnoses of perimenopause. This is a mistake that leaves so many young women in an identity crisis, feeling like they're growing old before their time, when in reality, the problem is viral—and manageable.

Infertility, Miscarriage, and Pregnancy Complications

There's a serious misconception growing among leaders in the thyroid health movement that hypothyroidism creates problems such as miscarriage, infertility, preeclampsia, and low birth weight. There's even a theory that a mother's hypothyroid can contribute to the development of ADHD for a child in the womb. This trend is heading to the point where in the coming years, anything pregnancy-related that's compromised on almost any level is going to be blamed on a mother's thyroid. Conventional doctors will be joining alternative medical communities in this thinking, and while it may seem advanced, it will distract from the truth about what's causing so much pain and suffering. Because if medical communities don't yet understand how thyroid illness really works, how can they make a solid link between it and pregnancy issues?

If you've heard that a hypothyroid was to blame for your miscarriage, struggle to conceive, or difficult pregnancy or childbirth and that explanation gave you peace, I don't mean to invalidate you in any way. There is still a very real explanation for what you've been through, and it's not your fault. Yes, it's very common to have a hypothyroid before or during pregnancy. That timing, however, does not make an underactive thyroid the cause of reproductive issues. Rather, a thyroid problem should be looked at as a clue or indicator of what's really going on—not the origin itself.

That true origin is something else entirely—something underfunded, ignored, and not researched enough. The same pathogen that's behind thyroid illness is behind so many reproductive struggles: EBV. Once again, this is an instance of your body getting the blame for your suffering when it's this pathogen that's really causing the problem. In reality, the thyroid is never responsible for miscarriages. Its radio-like frequencies sustain the reproductive system and growing baby, even when this gland is in trouble; the thyroid is so advanced that it's able to prevent pregnancy issues when its production of thyroid hormones is down. Plus, as we looked at earlier, to fill in for underproduction, the adrenals produce a hormone blend that mimics thyroid hormones (though it won't

show up on today's thyroid blood tests because its unique chemical composition doesn't create an *exact* match and is therefore undetectable for now).

The real trouble is when EBV targets the reproductive system. As you read earlier, partway through its second stage, EBV often enters the reproductive organs. This is what creates the circumstances for later fertility and pregnancy issues. By the time the virus reaches its third stage and enters the thyroid—often setting off hypothyroidism at this point—the uterus and/or ovaries have been battling the virus for some time, so problems start to showcase themselves at the same time the thyroid begins to act up. It just so happens that frequently, this is all happening during a woman's childbearing years, just when it can interfere the most.

Plus pregnancy and childbirth, with their influxes of hormones that feed EBV, can trigger a low-grade or dormant EBV infection to advance and multiply. Pregnancy also takes energy away from the immune system, making a woman more susceptible to EBV in her system. This means that a viral infection that hasn't caused symptoms in years could suddenly advance to the thyroid or wake from dormancy and become symptomatic and problematic when a woman becomes pregnant.

For example, a woman who had mono early in college may have had EBV that had advanced to her uterus by the time she graduated. As the virus nested there, it might have caused some uterine fibroids—though she would have had no way of knowing they were related to that mono freshman year. As the virus cycled between active periods and dormancy in her 20s, then perhaps moved on to the thyroid or beyond, she might have had other EBV symptoms come and go—ones such as weight gain, brain fog, joint pain, fatigue, hair loss, and dry, cracking skin—though again, there wouldn't be any evidence to connect this to her college days or her fibroids, so she wouldn't know it was all the same health story. Then, say she got pregnant in her early 30s and started to experience those earlier symptoms in full force—and also came close to losing the baby. A doctor might then run a blood panel on her and diagnose her with a hypothyroid, explaining that the low thyroid hormones were to blame for her symptoms and near miscarriage. In truth, it was the EBV the whole time.

So it's not the compromised thyroid *causing* the fertility issues; it's the virus in the reproductive system causing cysts, fibroids, inconsistent menstrual periods, fallopian tube obstruction, preeclampsia, and/or hidden and undetectable inflammation of the uterus that can interfere with a healthy conception and pregnancy.

That last issue, uterine inflammation, is behind so many mystery miscarriages. When EBV targets the uterus, it inflames the organ, creating a spasm that's impossible to detect and yet can interrupt a pregnancy. Miscarriages like this are most common among women with high viral loads and high concentrations of toxic heavy metals to feed the EBV. (Toxic heavy metals in the womb and passed along through sperm can also create problems for a developing baby. One example is ADHD—for the full explanation of this disorder, see the chapter dedicated to ADHD and autism in *Medical Medium*.)

Sometimes a woman gets hit with EBV symptoms after childbirth. As we looked at in Chapter 2, "Thyroid Virus Triggers," that's because the enormous supply of hormones that enter the bloodstream when a woman gives birth are fuel to Epstein-Barr virus cells. The amount of adrenaline that's released during this process is almost a lifetime's worth for someone who doesn't give birth—plenty to weaken the

immune system and launch EBV into high gear. The result is that a woman may experience crushing fatigue, depression, anxiety, weight gain, and brain fog that a doctor mistakenly diagnoses as postpartum depression, a thyroid issue, or even Lyme disease. (If a new mother is not overcome with an EBV infection, she may at least experience mild adrenal fatigue, listlessness, a bit of depression, and fatigue for a short period of time until she recovers from the hormone output.) EBV's more active, aggressive presence also means that a woman may have more difficulty trying to conceive or carry a baby to term with later pregnancies. None of the above means you need to avoid trying to conceive and have babies. Pregnancy and childbirth are beautiful, miraculous parts of life. You just need to give extra care to your adrenals and your overall health in order to stay a strong mom.

Another major contributing factor to many women's fertility issues is a low reproductive system "battery." This can occur on its own, with no viral activity in the body, or it can occur as a result of EBV draining the reproductive system of its energy and resources. In that case, it's best to work on lessening your viral load *and* recharging your battery. For more on this, see the chapter "Fertility and Our Future" in my book *Medical Medium Life-Changing Foods*.

Polycystic Ovarian Syndrome (PCOS)

As we just looked at, when EBV moves through the body, it may select the ovaries as a nesting place. There, the virus may prompt the creation of cysts as the immune system attempts to block off the growth of the virus, and the virus continues to live and grow inside them. As these cysts develop, they put a strain on the immune system, allowing EBV to move more quickly to

Stage Three, infection and disruption of the thyroid. That's why PCOS and thyroid issues occur side by side so often.

Weight gain is also commonly associated with PCOS. It doesn't occur *because* of PCOS, though, nor from a hormone imbalance—blaming weight gain on PCOS is merely an easy way for medical authorities to overlook the real issue. As we looked at in the weight gain section earlier in the chapter, it all comes down to the liver and lymphatic system. The reality is that in about half of PCOS cases, a woman does not experience weight gain. Those women who only have ovarian cyst issues with no weight issues are often younger, with livers that are relatively unburdened and lymphatic systems that are in better working shape. On the other hand, if a woman has lived for years with EBV, its waste matter, other toxins, and unproductive foods overloading her liver and causing backup in the lymphatic system, weight gain can be pronounced. It just so happens that at the same time, EBV is causing PCOS.

Breast Cancer

The true cause of breast cancer is the Epstein-Barr virus. When EBV is traveling from the liver to the thyroid, the lymphatic system tries to catch it in the chest area—and certain varieties of EBV, when caught here, will form tumors, cysts, or lesions. This is why breast cancer is often not limited to the breasts—it also commonly affects the armpits and lymph nodes.

MTHFR Gene Mutation

If you've been diagnosed with an MTHFR gene mutation, you have to keep in mind that no matter what you hear elsewhere, it's not technically a gene mutation. What's really occurring s that a viral infection of at least EBV (and, depending on the person, possibly an additional virus) has, over time, affected the liver, which has in turn affected the body's process of making and assimilating vitamin B_{12} and other key, critical nutrients. This elevates homocysteine levels, which triggers off a positive for MTHFR gene mutation in today's extremely unstable, new trendy test. Basically, it's just another (faulty) inflammation test like those we'll look at in "Great Mistake 4: Inflammation as Cause." Once your viral infection is under control or eliminated, the gene mutation test will change and show that you don't have a gene mutation—proof that it was never really a gene mutation to begin with. This is a charged topic, given that gene mutation diagnoses are on the rise, with excellent doctors and other practitioners investing a lot of time and energy in this now-confusing theory. You'll be hearing more from me about this in the future.

Injuries That Won't Heal

If an injury that seems like it should have gotten better a long time ago is still causing you pain and suffering, it may feel very disheartening if doctors can't determine why you're not feeling better and loved ones can't understand why you're not back to your old self. It's very common for people in this position to get the message that they're making up their pain, that they're holding on to an injury for attention or out of fear of getting better, or that they're not trying hard enough to heal. Don't let this thinking take you down! These are not the real explanations for your continued suffering.

When you're injured, the myelin sheaths covering the nerves in the area of the injury fray like strands of yarn, causing small nerve root hairs to come loose and hang or pop off the nerves. Injured nerves like these trigger an "alarm" hormone meant to bring your body's healing mechanisms to the rescue. When EBV is present in your system, though, it detects this hormone, too, and rushes over to take advantage and target the nerves. The disrupted root hairs give EBV the openings it needs to latch onto the nerves and keep them inflamed for a long period—sometimes years, if not addressed properly by taking care of your EBV.

If you're well into Stage Four of EBV, viral neurotoxins will also be released at record levels and cause nerve problems like never before—even without an accident or injury. As you've read about in previous symptoms, such as anxiety, tingles and numbness, and dizziness, high levels of these neurotoxins in the bloodstream create sensitized, allergic, inflamed nerves simply from proximity. The result is an extra difficult time healing when EBV is active in your system. Once you get rid of the virus, you can move forward.

Fibromyalgia

The aches, pains, tenderness, fatigue, and stiffness of fibromyalgia are a result of Stage Four EBV's neurotoxins creating chronic inflammation of both the central nervous system and nerves throughout the body. This can result in mild cracks, tears, and exposed root hairs that create sensitive spots on the nerves. Some aggressive varieties of EBV go so far as to bind onto these weak points, creating even more inflammation and pain.

Chronic Fatigue Syndrome (CFS), Chronic Fatigue Immune Dysfunction Syndrome (CFIDS), Myalgic Encephalomyelitis (ME), Systemic Exertion Intolerance Disease (SEID)

As medical communities try harder to understand this epic fatigue that was once labeled as laziness, this condition receives additional names. The truth is that CFS—or whichever name for it speaks to you—is neurological fatigue from an ongoing and chronic Stage Four EBV infection. Viral neurotoxins inflame and drain the central nervous system, creating an exhaustion that's often mistaken for adrenal fatigue (for more on the distinction, see the section "Fatigue" earlier in the chapter). In its more aggressive forms, the neurotoxins cause a mild encephalitis (which is undetectable by MRI or CT scan), which creates even heavier fatigue.

Eczema and Psoriasis

These skin conditions really all come down to undiscovered medical issues with the liver. They're not liver enzyme issues that a doctor will find on the rudimentary blood tests available, which don't detect much of what's going on with this complex organ. Rather, eczema and psoriasis occur due to a pathogen—usually EBV—in the liver that's feeding off of high levels of toxic copper there, plus old storage of DDT and other pesticides. When the virus feeds off these poisons, it releases a potent dermatoxin, which floats up to the skin, causing severe rashes, flaking, cracking, irritation, and itching.

Ideally, the liver would filter out these dermatoxins like other debris, and the intestinal tract and kidneys would send them out of the body. However, when EBV is overloading the liver and the rest of the body, normal detox processes get interrupted, which is why these toxins end up trying to leave through the skin. The worse off the liver is, the worse the eczema or psoriasis, as the liver's impeded function means more dermatoxins escape. People with more eczema or psoriasis are also more prone to experience hair loss on the scalp.

Lupus

Medical communities have not yet been able to identify what causes this inflammatory condition, so it's been mistakenly labeled as autoimmune. That's not how it works at all—lupus is not evidence of the immune system going haywire and targeting the body. The true cause of lupus is EBV. Essentially, lupus is an allergic reaction to the virus's waste matter: dermatoxins (hence the skin issues so commonly associated with lupus), neurotoxins, byproduct, and viral corpses. When too much of this sludge builds up over time, then by Stage Three of EBV, the body can become hypersensitive to it, resulting in various symptoms of inflammation. This also elevates homocysteine levels, triggering false positives on gene mutation tests. (When you clean up EBV, those gene mutation tests go back to normal.)

Because lupus begins in Stage Three, when EBV is also targeting the thyroid, anyone who has lupus also has a compromised thyroid, whether they know it or not.

Multiple Sclerosis (MS)

The Epstein-Barr virus is the hidden cause of MS. There are two types of EBV that result in this diagnosis: (1) In this type of EBV, a person exhibits neurological symptoms such as weak legs, weak arms, mild tremors, and severe tingles and numbness. These are the result of EBV neurotoxins inflaming various nerves in the body. It's commonly diagnosed as MS (or Lyme disease), though no lesions will show on medical scans. (2) This other type of EBV reaches the brain, where it causes lesions, mild forms of encephalitis, and very similar symptoms as the previous type. If you've been diagnosed with brain lesions, do not fear them; hundreds of thousands of people walk around with various lesions in their brains, from small to large, and they continue to live their lives. In many cases, the symptoms that go along with this type of EBV are not from the lesions themselves; they're still from those EBV neurotoxins.

Because MS occurs in Stage Four of EBV, people with this condition also have a thyroid problem, whether diagnosed or not. The best way to deal with either type of MS diagnosis—and with the thyroid issue—is to deal with the EBV at hand and to strengthen the nervous system. (For much more on MS, see its chapter in *Medical Medium*.)

Lyme Disease

Depending on what doctor you visit, certain symptoms can be diagnosed as MS, fibromyalgia, chronic fatigue syndrome, RA, amyotrophic lateral sclerosis (ALS), parasitical infection, lupus, or Lyme disease—because these conditions are all virus-caused, and so the lines often blur between these labels. That's right: as I exposed in my first book, Lyme disease is viral—not bacterial. I don't say this to negate the progress made in medical communities that's come from acknowledging the many people who suffer from Lyme symptoms and making efforts to offer them answers. The next step will be for medical research to uncover that the cause of Lyme disease symptoms is viral—bacteria only happen to be present. Most people's Lyme symptoms are caused by EBV, though all other viruses in the herpetic family can also cause them, including HHV-6 all the way up through the undiscovered HHV-9, HHV-10, HHV-11, and HHV-12. Surprise! If reading this puts you in shock, go check out the Lyme disease chapter in *Medical Medium* for answers to all of your questions.

If you've already read that chapter, you might have noticed that its Lyme trigger list looked very similar to the thyroid virus triggers in Chapter 2 of this book. That's because, once again, both Lyme and thyroid conditions are viral—so there's a lot of overlap in what triggers their symptoms.

Rheumatoid Arthritis (RA)

This swelling, pain, stiffness, and sometimes deformity of the joints is not an autoimmune disorder—that explanation for RA couldn't be further from the truth. The body does not become confused and start attacking your joints. Rather, there's a specific variety of EBV that gets into connective tissue, joints, and ligaments in its fourth stage, causing inflammation that's evidence of your body trying to hold the invader at bay. Swelling of the knuckles, cervical spine, and the like is an indication that the immune system is fighting to keep the virus from burrowing deeper and causing permanent damage to nerves and tissue. In its milder forms, this may display itself as mystery aches and pains. In its advanced forms, people experience severe joint swelling and a diagnosis of RA.

Connective Tissue Disorders (including Ehlers-Danlos Syndrome)

These conditions are caused by a variety of EBV in Stage Four (sometimes Stage Three) that's feeding off of different toxins in the liver, including old DDT and other pesticides, mercury, and some solvents. Many of these can be passed down through a family line, inherited from past generations. As the virus thrives on this fuel blend, it releases both neurotoxins and a specific connective tissue toxin, a combination that weakens connective tissue and inflames nerves at the same time. Because this is a late-stage EBV condition, it's a sign that you have thyroid issues, too, though it's not a thyroid *symptom*.

Sarcoidosis

Some varieties of EBV are less concentrated on the central nervous system and instead make their focus the lymphatic system and organs. In these cases, as the virus advances to later phases and stages, many virus cells also stay behind to attack and inflame lymph nodes around the lungs, heart, liver, and neck, creating swelling and scar tissue throughout the lymphatic system and in and around the organs. This gets to the point of sarcoidosis by Stage Four of the virus—which means that sarcoidosis is an indication that someone has also developed a thyroid condition (Stage Three EBV) by this point, though again, it's not thyroid-caused.

Pulmonary Fibrosis, Cystic Fibrosis, Interstitial Lung Disease

These conditions that commonly affect the lungs are all caused by EBV and antibiotic-resistant strains of EBV's cofactor, *Streptococcus* bacteria—the same culprit behind so many common issues, including chronic urinary tract infections (UTIs) and strep throat. Staying clear of eggs, dairy, wheat, and pork is critical with these conditions.

Hypoglycemia and Type 2 Diabetes

It's very common for type 2 diabetes to accompany a thyroid condition, because EBV, other toxins, and a high-fat diet put a strain on the liver that makes it sluggish or stagnant and unable to store glucose as glycogen to protect the pancreas, which you rely on for insulin. At the same time, as the adrenals overcompensate for the thyroid, all that excess adrenaline scorches the pancreas, further compromising its ability to produce the insulin you need. As a result, you experience blood sugar imbalances. (For a full explanation of hypoglycemia and type 2 diabetes, see their dedicated chapter in my first book.)

Acid Reflux

When someone experiences heartburn, half the problem is in the stomach and the other half is in the liver. That's because acid reflux actually occurs from low hydrochloric acid (a beneficial acid) in the stomach—which commonly happens when the liver is dysfunctional from EBV and so under-produces bile to aid with digestion. As a result, bad acids in the stomach rise.

When they go up the esophagus, the sensation is heartburn.

It's unknown to medical research and science that not only can EBV contribute to acid reflux; the condition also gets in the way of thyroid healing. When people have elevated levels of unproductive acids in their stomachs due to low hydrochloric acid (good acid), those bad acids tend to rise up the esophagus during sleep, going all the way to the throat, where they outgas ammonia, which can seep directly into the thyroid and inhibit the gland's healing.

Streptococcus

Because strep bacteria is a cofactor to EBV, it prospers when the virus does. This is why people with thyroid issues are no strangers to sinus problems, bladder sensitivities, urinary tract infections (UTIs), bacterial vaginosis, small intestinal bacterial overgrowth (SIBO), IBS, acne, and sore throats—all of which are strep-related.

Celiac Disease

Celiac is not an autoimmune condition, nor is it limited to a sensitivity to gluten. Rather, wheat gluten is one trigger to this inflammation of the intestinal tract, which is in fact caused by EBV's cofactor strep. Strep's other favorite foods to find in the gut are eggs, dairy products, and corn alongside biofilm, neurotoxins, viral casings, other EBV waste, and toxic heavy metals dumping from the liver into the intestinal tract. These items give strep the fuel to prosper and irritate.

Raynaud's Syndrome

This skin discoloration occurs as a result of a liver partially clogged by EBV and its waste matter that's backing up into the bloodstream. In most cases of Raynaud's, someone has had a longstanding infection of EBV, since childhood, and while much of the virus has moved on to the thyroid and beyond, some of the virus has remained in the liver, causing long-term problems. When the blood fills with these viral toxins, it gets thick, causing blood toxicity, and the result is poor circulation to the extremities—which causes them to become discolored. Many people with Raynaud's also experience a bit of tingling or sometimes even numbness, because the sludge that backs up into the bloodstream has neurotoxins in it.

Cushing's Syndrome

Cushing's is understood by medical communities to be an adrenal dysfunction, and that's true to a degree. What isn't understood is the full underlying cause: When you've had a thyroid condition from EBV for a long time, your adrenals have spent years in overdrive, trying to fill in as the thyroid hormone creators and balancers. An EBV-strained liver, too, puts further stress on the adrenals. On top of this adrenal strain, people with Cushing's have typically also encountered massive stress in life and faced other factors, such as poor diet, that weakened the adrenals. Pushed to the max from these multiple sources, the adrenals become dysfunctional, and the result is weight gain in certain areas of the body, along with skinnier arms and legs. Though you may hear otherwise, true Cushing's usually hits when people are in their mid-40s to mid-60s, due to the time it takes for the adrenals to become so imbalanced.

Hepatitis C

This chronic inflammation of the liver is caused by EBV creating scar tissue in the organ—a discovery that medical research and science are going to land on pretty soon. Because of the years it takes for EBV to create this disruptive scarring, by the time it's turned into hepatitis C, other EBV cells have already advanced to the thyroid or beyond—meaning that those with hepatitis C are also dealing with compromised thyroids. This length of time it takes to develop is also why hepatitis C commonly presents in older people.

Plantar Fasciitis

When EBV releases large amounts of neurotoxins throughout the body, those neurotoxins disperse and settle on weak nerves in the body. If someone was once highly active on her or his feet, or once injured her or his feet or ankles, whether from dancing, athletics, a turned ankle, or an accident, the neurotoxins find these sensitive nerves almost as if they're targeting them, resulting in inflammation and pain in nerves such as the tibial and the sciatic. For many, plantar fasciitis arises long after an initial injury, because it could be that an injury happened years before a person had an active, late-stage EBV infection.

Parathyroid Disease

Though the four tiny glands known as the parathyroid function separately from the thyroid, when they develop problems, the culprit is the same as with thyroid disease: EBV. Together, these glands, which are each about the size of a shelled sunflower seed, are responsible for keeping calcium levels balanced in the body—basically, they regulate calcium levels in the bloodstream. Parathyroid disease usually means that one or more of these glands have become inflamed, enlarged, calcified, cystic, or tumorous due to an EBV infection (medical research and science don't yet know this is the cause), consequently throwing off the calcium production and monitoring system of the body.

There is a tie between the thyroid and the parathyroid: When the body is creating thyroid nodules to try to wall off EBV cells, the parathyroid becomes involved. Remember, nodules are calcium prisons—so the parathyroid may respond to this nodule formation by overproducing parathyroid hormone (to assist the body with making the nodules), or in some cases under-producing (to protect calcium reserves), depending on your individual needs. When the parathyroid is overactive in this circumstance, it usually doesn't show up on tests, because the extra calcium goes to immediate use.

The parathyroid also receives physical protection from the thyroid—these glands need to be shielded from the sun, and the thyroid's wing structure does that shielding.

Like thyroid issues, parathyroid issues don't necessarily show up on tests, so there are people walking around with undiagnosed hyperparathyroidism. One common cause of this condition is EBV leaving the thyroid at the end of Stage Three and beginning to target the central nervous system. At this point, the brain starts to require more electrolytes to support neurotransmitter function and electrical impulses, which triggers the parathyroid to signal for more calcium to support this extra electrical function needed for the central nervous system to deal with the EBV. The virus can also target the parathyroid itself, throwing it into dysfunction and directly causing parathyroid disease. This all remains undiscovered by medical research and science.

WHY WOMEN?

Why is it that many of the symptoms and conditions you just read about affect women in greater numbers than men? Why do we so frequently hear about thyroid problems and mysterious chronic illness as a women's issue?

To begin with, some of that perception is askew. Historically, there was greater stigma for men to admit to physical challenge. In the 1940s and 1950s, as women were visiting the doctor describing their health struggles, men, too, were experiencing an outbreak of depression, anxiety, mood swings, excessive sweating, body temperature fluctuations, brain fog, heart palpitations, and the like. However, stoicism had a high value for men. They'd grown up with the message that they had to be strong and stable, and so many of them stayed away from the doctor and kept quiet about their symptoms, creating the illusion that only women were suffering. Then, once women's symptoms had created enough of a stir in medical communities to get the widespread label of menopause, men's similar symptoms became even more stigmatized. Now a man would not only feel hesitant to admit to "weakness"; doing so also had the potential to embarrass him with the association that he was going through his own "change of life."

Even though it hasn't been as apparent, EBV has affected men greatly, and there's no shame in it. Liver issues, weight gain, restless legs, hypertension, high cholesterol, and constipation are just a few examples of those symptoms you can probably identify in at least one man in your life. Prostate cancer, too, originates from EBV.

Still, there is a lot of truth to the observation that women are up against chronic symptoms such as thyroid issues at higher rates than men. Much of this has to do with a woman's reproductive cycle. Each month, her system puts a tremendous amount of energy and resources into preparing her body for the possibility of a baby. When a woman is menstruating, 80 percent of her body's active immune system and reserves go toward renewing her womb— which significantly cuts the energy her body has to ward off illness at that time. And during ovulation, 40 percent of her body's immune system and reserves go toward the process—once again leaving the door open for illness to take advantage. Plus, her production of cortisol and adrenaline both go up at these times, sending EBV fuel into her bloodstream. This all means that twice a month, women become more susceptible to health threats such as EBV. It's why women often come down with a cold, flu, migraine, or sore throat right before or during menstruation—because their immune systems drop.

Not to mention that these days, women live with more expectations than ever. With pressure to hold down careers, run their households, please their partners, lend sympathy and empathy to friends, care for their families, and look good while doing it, most women end up with practically 10, 20, or 30 jobs. On top of the physical and mental toll this takes, the awareness, intuition, and compassion required to keep all this going can also be a drain if there's no chance to restore. It's very easy to become run-down with all of this going on, and a run-down immune system is one of EBV's favorite avenues of advancement.

This means that women can't get away with not caring for themselves. If you're a woman, and you've felt you needed approval to make your health a priority, consider this your permission slip. Especially during menstruation, ovulation, pregnancy, and recovery from childbirth, take the measures you need to stay balanced. It's the best thing you can do for those who rely on you—too much hangs in the balance otherwise.

No matter who you are, you deserve to acknowledge any health problems you've faced with the mind-set that it's not a poor reflection on you. If you're a man, remember: The symptoms and conditions you've read about in this chapter are not solely women's issues; EBV is an equal opportunity pathogen. You deserve self-care, too. With EBV exposed for what it is, you can see your struggles in a whole new light.

CHAPTER 6

Thyroid Cancer

My introduction to cancer came at age four, at the same time that I first received my gift from Spirit. I was seated at the family dinner table when Spirit appeared to me, instructing me to inform my grandmother that she had lung cancer. Though I didn't know what the term meant, I repeated it, much to the shock of everyone at the table. The doctor soon confirmed that the revelation was true.

Afterward, I asked Spirit how it had happened. Why had my grandmother gotten cancer? Spirit answered that it was a combination of a virus, EBV, plus a variety of toxins in the form of heavy metals, DDT and other pesticides, solvents, plastics, and petroleum. The words were foreign to me at that young age, though I could tell they were serious. Since then—for the entire time I've had this gift—I've taken cancer personally. Over the decades, I've helped countless people who were battling cancer to find answers, safety, and healing.

I've been asked why I haven't addressed cancer in my previous books. In fact, the topic of cancer does show up in both books, most notably in *Medical Medium Life-Changing Foods*, where dozens of foods are noted for their cancer-fighting properties, with targeted healing foods for specific forms of cancer—including thyroid cancer. I understand why people still want more. Cancer is a big and scary topic, and it remains a mystery to medical research and science. The answers aren't out there about why it even exists or how to protect yourself and your loved ones, so people are left with a void.

With every book, I want to include as much healing information as I possibly can. I set out to give you every possible insight at once, and then I always come up against the reality: that it's just one book, and I can't fit in everything there is to say. Until now, there simply hasn't been room to address cancer in more detail. I believe it's finally time to change that.

THE NOT-SO-DISTANT PAST

You'll hear from other sources that cancer has always been part of our human history. Going back 500 years, 1,000 years, even going back to ancient times, these sources say, cancer has gotten in the way of life. You'll be told that cancer can be found in mummies, and one day, you'll even be told that cancer was discovered in a caveman found preserved in ice for tens of thousands of years.

The truth is that real, malignant cancer is a comparatively recent development. While the tumors of old could be life-threatening if they grew in such a way that they impeded organ function, they weren't caused by cancer cells; they were benign. When the ancient Greeks used the word that eventually led to our English word *cancer*, they weren't referring to what we mean today when we say "cancer." Theirs was a blanket term for all disease, when someone was ailing, not recovering, and even dying without explanation. Tumors—non-cancerous tumors—made up only a tiny fraction of that definition. The tumors of the day formed from old scar tissue from flesh wounds and from toxic heavy metals saturating living tissue. Real, malignant cancer's true origins only go back to the Industrial Revolution.

Why are we told otherwise? Why are we led to believe that cancer is practically prehistoric? Because if we believe that cancer has been with us since the beginning of humankind, then we'll think that a predisposition toward it is written into our genes, and therefore we're the ones who should take the blame for it. If we're convinced that we create cancer within ourselves or that cancer is our fault because we're frail human beings, we won't look harder for the answers we're not supposed to know.

Well, you deserve answers—so let's get rid of the mystery around thyroid cancer.

THE THYROID CANCER VIRUS

Ninety-eight percent of the time, cancer is caused by a virus and at least one type of toxin. There are many viruses that can be involved with cancer; EBV is one of them, and in combination with toxins, it's the virus responsible for thyroid cancer. (EBV is also responsible for breast cancer, liver cancer, almost all lung cancer, pancreatic cancer, colon cancer, prostate cancer, women's reproductive cancers, leukemia, and many more.)

It's easy to think that a mother and daughter who look alike and sound alike and both develop thyroid cancer in their lifetimes get that same cancer because of genes. That's what we're supposed to think, because it keeps us from investigating outside sources.

While of course facial features and vocal chords are genetic, disease isn't. Here's the real equation: **Virus + Toxins = Cancer**

When a particular virus has the right fuel in the form of particular toxins, cancer can result. Notice how genes aren't part of that at all? What medical communities interpret as genetics with cancer susceptibility is really the passing along of viruses and toxins from generation to generation, or exposure within a family to the same viruses and toxins because the family lives together. That mother and daughter could have both inherited EBV through the family line, and then, during the daughter's childhood, both could have been exposed to nasty toxins that fed the virus.

To examine how the Epstein-Barr virus became part of the cancer equation, let's touch back on the historical development of EBV. First, the Industrial Revolution came along, and with it, the development of brand-new, heavy-metal-laden chemical compounds that began to pollute our world and our bodies. EBV would feed off of these poisons to try to protect us from them like the good, loyal virus it still was, and in processing them, the virus cells would essentially remanufacture the poisons into more toxic form, releasing them in order to protect itself into whatever tissue surrounded it—whether in the liver, lungs, pancreas, breasts, thyroid, or elsewhere. Once eliminated as EBV byproduct, these remanufactured poisons could serve as food again to the virus. This would happen continually, with only the strongest virus cells—ones that could tolerate the ever-stronger poisons—surviving and multiplying.

When EBV was first morphing like this, it wasn't yet cancerous. Benign tumors could form from the dead human tissue killed off by EBV's poisonous remanufactured byproduct; for the most part, that was it. (Malignant EBV tumors were still extremely rare. Those that did form were a result of the very first mutated strain of EBV that came into contact with early, experimental chemical compounds.) What this time period really did was set the stage for certain strains of EBV to go cancerous eventually, when they encountered the right fuel.

As the decades passed and we entered the second half of the 1800s, the virus grew even stronger. Then came more industrial chemical creations, this time the experimental fungicides, herbicides, and antibiotics of the late 1800s that took EBV to a new level, forcing the virus to mutate so that it was one no longer beneficial to our bodies. With these new chemical compounds as fuel, EBV's toxic waste was more poisonous than ever before in its history. When this viral byproduct saturated the living tissue of whichever part of the body it was in at a given time—for example, the thyroid—the formation of keloids and benign tumors from damaged, scarred tissue and dead human cells became more common. EBV, at the same time, was mutating in order to tolerate its own remanufactured, poisonous waste. It was only out for itself now.

As we moved into the 20th century, certain varieties of EBV became signature to creating cancer. And through the last 100-plus years, these EBV strains have continued to mutate as they consume more advanced, newer brews of toxins.

HOW THYROID CANCER FORMS

When someone contracts one of the mutated strains of EBV that can cause cancer, the strain keeps mutating inside the body if it has the right fuel in the form of toxins. The virus takes in the toxins in its path and goes through that remanufacturing process, releasing poisons that are stronger than when they went in, almost like the trial-and-error synthesis process that goes into chemical companies' creation of new, potent chemical compounds. This probably sounds similar to the Chapter 3 description of how neurotoxins and dermatoxins are produced, and it is. The difference is that cancer-causing EBV strains tend to produce fewer neurotoxins and dermatoxins than some other EBV varieties; instead, they're geared to remanufacture toxins into more overall cell-damaging poisons. If the virus is in the thyroid at this point, the remanufactured poisons will saturate the area of the gland where the virus cells are located, damaging thyroid tissue. The virus will consume the dead tissue cells that are filled with remanufactured poisons, and much of the virus will start to die off from the toxicity—in fact, someone's viral load inside the thyroid could reduce 50 to 70 percent at this stage.

Another cycle will begin. The EBV cells that survive will be the ones best equipped to handle poisons. They'll feed on any old or new toxins in that person's body. Plus their viral byproduct—this time even more potent after another round of reprocessing—will saturate the thyroid tissue again, killing off some of the healthy thyroid cells, and the virus will consume these poison-saturated tissue cells, too. The EBV cells that can't tolerate the increased toxicity will die off, and the new round of survivors will be even stronger than before.

A third cycle will start. This time, as the virus resynthesizes and remanufactures another batch of poisons, it again saturates adjacent thyroid tissue and consumes the toxic, dead thyroid cells that result. Instead of a normal die-off, like the virus cells of the previous cycles that took place six months to two years earlier, the virus cells that are poisoned this time reach their mutation capacity. As a last-ditch method of survival when no longer able to mutate, these dying virus cells produce an enzymatic chemical compound that transforms them into living cancer cells. Now, instead of being on the brink of death, they have an afterlife.

With new structures, these cells consume the remanufactured-poison-saturated thyroid cells in order to reproduce and multiply, this time as cancer. As they do this, the cancer cells will in turn release a new enzymatic biochemical into nearby thyroid tissue, slowly morphing those human cells into cancer cells as well.

Both the formerly viral cancer cells and the formerly human cancer cells have life to them, and they group together to survive. In these clusters, they need food. A process of angiogenesis occurs, where tiny blood vessels form—similar to the tiny veins in a leaf—to draw up nutrients past the microscopic membrane holding the cluster of cancer cells together. (Angiogenesis as a concept has been discovered by medical science and research, though the specifics we're looking at in this chapter are not yet known.)

Meanwhile, there are still active EBV cells in the thyroid that haven't turned cancerous. They're continuing to cycle through consuming and re-consuming toxins, and their waste matter can continue to kill off living thyroid tissue. The vessels of the cancerous cell mass will suck up both the remanufactured poisons and the dead human cells as fuel, allowing a malignant thyroid tumor or cyst to form—and then to grow and expand.

IT TAKES TWO

Let's be perfectly clear that EBV does not automatically translate to thyroid cancer. First of all, only some mutated strains in EBV Groups 4 and 5 can form cancer cells. Secondly, a particularly strong brew of toxins needs to be part of the equation, too. As you could see in the process we just examined, EBV needed fuel at every step of the way in order to advance to the point of cancer.

We're not supposed to think too much about the toxins involved in cancer. We're not supposed to know we inherit them. Instead, as I said, we're supposed to think cancer is genetic. If it's genetic, then it's our fault, and if it's our fault, then no one else will pay the price. Think about mesothelioma, a cancer caused by asbestos exposure (one of the rare few cancers that does not involve a virus). When the cause of mesothelioma came to light, companies were forced to put together a multibillion-dollar fund for patients and families affected by the cancer. That's just one industrial-borne toxin. Now imagine if the industries responsible for the production of all the various toxins that feed EBV were exposed. Billions alone would need to go into researching EBV and its mutations. It would be catastrophic—class-action lawsuits would follow, dozens of multi-*trillion*-dollar funds would need to be established, and industries would pay the price for over 150 years of cancer.

So instead of the truth coming out about how various cancers develop, we're told that we create it with our DNA or even our thoughts. Medical research and science focus on genes being responsible for cancer and how to treat cancer once it's already formed, and the process of how cancer actually starts stays in the dark.

Now you know the truth, though, and that truth involves toxins. So many variables affect how an EBV-caused (or any virus-caused) cancer forms and develops. Does someone have more dioxins in the body? More heavy metals, more pesticides, more pharmaceuticals? What kinds? What poisons were inherited through the family line? Then there's the virus—what strain is it? How mutated? If someone has fewer toxins and a strain of the virus that's less aggressive, their cancer may not be as pernicious, and if it's otherwise, the cancer may develop much more quickly. And there's the immune system to consider—is it compromised, or still going strong? If we were to make great strides in understanding cancer as a society, this is where medical research and science would focus.

A FORMULA FOR HEALING

The virus-plus-toxins formula may sound frightening. Don't let it worry you. It's much less frightening than not knowing how or why cancer plagues us.

Say you learn about a 90-year-old who smoked for 70 years and never developed lung cancer. While he might have had plenty of other negative health effects from smoking, cancer wasn't one of them. Then you think about someone who did develop lung cancer and never smoked a day in his life, though was exposed to another type of toxic brew. What distinguished the two? Until now, you probably would have said that the answer was a mystery and most likely came down to genetics. In light of this chapter, you can say that the one who didn't get cancer was the one without a virus.

And that knowledge gives you control in your own life—a wildly better option than living in fear. Whether you'd like to prevent thyroid cancer or deal with thyroid cancer you already have, you now know the steps to take: (1) lower your viral load, and (2) eliminate toxins from your body. This book gives you the power to do both.

Now, to give you an even fuller picture of your health-care story, let's look at how thyroid blood tests really work.

CHAPTER 7

Thyroid Guess Tests

Women have been trying for decades to make themselves heard about their symptoms. It hasn't been an easy process. For so long, they were made to feel like so many of the health challenges we looked at in Chapter 5 were all in their heads. Then finally, as medical communities began to identify thyroid issues as widespread, testing for those issues also reached mainstream medicine. This has offered validation to so many patients who receive proof with test results that there's something amiss in their bodies.

On the other hand, what if you're one of those women (or men) whose test results come back "normal"? There's been a long-standing practice where traditional doctors take all their thyroid cues from a patient's TSH (thyroid-stimulating hormone, also called thyrotropin) levels. They want to see those readings in the normal range of 0.5 to 5.0, and if they are, then these doctors go by what they've been taught: that a patient's thyroid is fine. It can feel like such a blow to hear that everything looks as it should when you know something's wrong.

Now we've got doctors who are trying to investigate a little deeper. They see many patients whose TSH levels come back normal despite a range of symptoms that seem to indicate otherwise, so they're trying to get a more comprehensive sense of thyroid performance by testing for

free T4 and free T3 at the same time. It's progress in the sense that women are being taken seriously now more than ever.

Even with this awakening, though, we're stuck in the antique-shopping phase of thyroid testing, because every thyroid test out there is built around the antiquated assumption that the problem with people's health is an ailing thyroid. And as you know well by now, a thyroid that's in trouble is not the problem itself; it's an indication of something much bigger: an Epstein-Barr viral load. If the latest information you're hearing or reading out there says otherwise, the source should be considered a throwback to the Dark Ages or even the time of the dinosaurs and a relic of outmoded thinking.

Until medical communities wake up to the fact that EBV is the real culprit behind thyroid issues—and not just a sidekick to other factors mistakenly regarded as the instigators of people's poor health—thyroid testing will remain limited in its helpfulness. Even as new, groundbreaking thyroid tests come to the table, which they will, they won't be enough. Research can come up with the best, most state-of-the-art methods for testing the performance of the thyroid gland, and they will completely miss the point. What doctors and labs really need are more advanced tests for EBV— tests that track where the virus is in a person's body, its path of travel through that individual's system, its levels in various organs and glands, and how it feeds and mutates.

So the premise of testing thyroid hormone production itself already falls short. These tests misdirect health-care professionals and patients, making everyone focus on one effect of the virus (impairment of the thyroid), rather than the much bigger picture that it's a virus *causing* that damage and wreaking havoc elsewhere in the body at the same time. For this reason, I won't go into great depth here on the specific tests.

THYROID HORMONE TESTS

That said, tests such as those for T4, T3, and thyroid-stimulating hormone (TSH) are what we have right now, and they are pieces of the puzzle. If you and your doctor interpret them with the mind-set that they're indicators of a virus affecting the thyroid gland, rather than the thyroid becoming weak and letting you down, then they can put you on the right track—if your tests come back indicating abnormalities in thyroid performance.

As I said, many enlightened doctors and patients have begun to notice that these tests can come back in the normal range even when every other sign points to something amiss. Here's why: The accuracy of these blood tests is, unfortunately, inconsistent—that's why I call them *guess tests*. To begin with, thyroid hormone readings can vary widely depending on the time of day and the patient's stress levels. It's much like the "white coat syndrome" many people experience when they walk into a doctor's office and get their blood pressure taken. Just sitting there under observation can get your palms sweaty and raise your blood pressure above normal levels, throwing off the accuracy of the readings.

In the same way, sitting in a lab or exam room about to have your blood drawn can get your adrenals pumping, which completely changes your blood chemistry—because suddenly, adrenaline (also known as epinephrine) and cortisol (also known as hydrocortisone), both steroids, flood the bloodstream in preparation for fight-or-flight, disrupting homeostasis in the process. These high adrenaline and cortisol levels can make it look on a blood test like you're producing more than enough of the thyroid-related steroids T4, T3, and TSH—whether you truly are or not. Or adrenaline and cortisol may be saturating your brain and putting your pituitary gland, which produces TSH, into overdrive—again, throwing off blood-test results from what they'd look like normally.

Even if the sight of a needle doesn't bother you at all, a disruption of homeostasis could still be affecting your blood chemistry. If you're someone who experiences chronic stress, then you may live with constant elevated adrenaline and cortisol, or, as we looked at earlier, these levels may be high from compensating for your underactive thyroid, or you may have adrenal fatigue. With adrenal fatigue, the adrenal glands can produce adrenaline and cortisol erratically, sometimes flooding the bloodstream and sometimes holding back. In this case, your adrenals may be overactive when you're getting your blood drawn even if the doctor's office is your favorite place in the world, and so, again, the results can be inaccurate.

I've seen people get a thyroid blood test one week, go back to get blood taken a week later for another purpose, and have the thyroid profiles on each come back with completely different numbers. Assessing the results of just one thyroid test is too limiting; it means that doctors can unknowingly miss if a patient has a thyroid condition. With blood pressure, many doctors and nurse practitioners have learned that the best way to deal with inaccurate measurements is to take a few blood pressure readings over the course of an appointment and average them. A similar approach would help with thyroid testing—although what it would really take is a thyroid test once a day for 30 days, and then an average at the end of the month.

This would be more helpful, though it still wouldn't solve everything, because the tests themselves are antiquated. A few decades from now, hopefully medical communities will finally catch on to the true, viral cause of thyroid disease, and the testing will be better. Until then, health-care professionals and patients deal with thyroid tests that are too broad in range and not attuned to the subtle hormonal shifts that can signal a thyroid condition. The hormone guess tests are so unstable that it would almost be more accurate to make a fist for 10 seconds, release it, and see if it took more than three seconds for color to come back to your palm as an indication of a thyroid problem.

Millions of women unknowingly walk around with hypothyroids that wouldn't register on today's tests. Sometimes it takes months or years of living with an underactive thyroid for it to progress to the point that a lab can detect it. In the meantime, a person must live with worsening health due to the virus's progression—and no answers. While we can pretend everything is fine, that won't get anyone better.

None of which is to say that you should write off thyroid tests. You simply need the background above so you can interpret the results with perspective. If you're going in for thyroid testing, ask to be tested for TSH, free T4, free T3, and thyroid antibodies.

Reverse T3 testing is currently a fad that's not worth dwelling on. While it does reflect genuine problems, it can pick up on so many at once that it's hard to know what any result means. It's fine to have your doctor order the test; it just may not help you pinpoint to a reliable degree.

THYROID ANTIBODIES TESTS

Thyroid antibodies tests deserve some extra attention here, because out of the thyroid tests, these are the closest to picking up on viral activity. Again, though, it's all about perspective. Currently, medical communities consider the antibodies detected in these tests to be autoantibodies (also called antithyroid antibodies and antimicrosomal antibodies)—that is, antibodies your immune system creates to go after your own thyroid tissue. The antibodies are taken as evidence that your body is attacking your thyroid, and you end up with an autoimmune diagnosis. In reality, this is not what's happening; that interpretation is based completely on assumption. When scientists first discovered the antibody activity and couldn't figure out why it was happening, it was a convenient theory to say that the body must be malfunctioning. Trouble is, neither conventional nor alternative medical communities have yet moved on from that theory. It remains undeveloped science.

Remember, your body does not attack itself. The antibodies that show up in tests such as the thyroid peroxidase (TPO) test are, in fact, your saving grace. They are not going after your thyroid—they do not cause damage to the gland on any level. These antibodies are created by your immune system to target the true troublemaker: EBV.

Part of what confuses medical communities is that medical research and science have not yet discovered the thyroid's personalized immune system that we looked at in Chapter 5, "Your Symptoms and Conditions—Explained."

The special lymphocytes we talked about, which are not yet catalogued, are assigned to the thyroid area, like soldiers that guard the thyroid. Though they're temporarily led away from the thyroid during the transition from Stage Two to Stage Three, the thyroid—a highly intelligent gland— sends out an emergency signal for the specialized lymphocytes to return once the thyroid realizes it's under attack. Once back, the lymphocytes work symbiotically with the antibodies your immune system produces, allowing these antibodies into the thyroid so that the antibodies can attack the EBV there and get it out of your body. The confusion here is that medical communities see the antibody activity and think it means that's the source of the problem. This is not accurate. Your special lymphocytes and these antibodies are working together to defend you.

So when looking at the results of any thyroid antibodies tests, remind yourself that if antibodies show up, they're due to viral activity in your thyroid—not a mistaken response by your body— and if antibodies don't show up, this doesn't mean EBV isn't present in the thyroid. Like the others, it's a test that's still in progress. Unlike with thyroid hormone tests, it's not blood chemistry that can throw off antibodies tests. Rather, the antibodies tests' weakness is that they are not yet broad enough or sensitive enough to detect smaller amounts of antibodies. When EBV is in an early phase in the thyroid, your immune system hasn't yet made use of all its bells and whistles, so the antibody activity may not be enough to register on lab work.

Plus, there are so many varieties of EBV, with mutations continuing to develop, and this diversity means that there is also diversity in the possible antibody reactions and antibody creations they induce, with certain antibodies geared toward these mutations that are not on blood labs' radar. Current tests only pick up some of those reactions and creations. Translation: You may well have antibodies in your system that test results don't show. These are antibody varieties that are literally "off the chart" because they are uncharted territory—they haven't been discovered, so blood labs don't look for them. If a blood lab doesn't know an antibody exists, it's not going to be commissioned to search for it. It takes funding and authorization to look outside the box of what's known—although you don't need a lesson from me on red tape and regulations. I'm sure one way or another, you're plenty familiar with these.

YOUR OWN THYROID EXPERT

Given that these scientific methods of diagnosis are still in development, when it comes to determining if you have a thyroid illness, you are your own best expert. If your test results don't give you any insights, know that if you are experiencing any of the late-stage symptoms we looked at in Chapter 5, they can be major indications that your thyroid has already been targeted by EBV and continues to be affected even as the EBV advances through your system.

Above all, remember that your thyroid is only one part of what's going on with your health. Though all of the medical focus on thyroid testing can make it seem like the opposite—and past test results may have made you feel like you were either making up your problem, or like your thyroid was in terrible shape and you were somehow to blame—don't let it get you down. Today's thyroid guess tests are not, ultimately, about getting to the root of your health problem and offering you answers. They're about determining whether someone should go on thyroid medication—a topic we'll cover in the next chapter.

CHAPTER 8

Thyroid Medication

For centuries, there was a popular concept that if a part of your body was ailing, you treated it by consuming that same body part of an animal. If, for example, your leg were diseased, you might eat a leg of lamb in an attempt to bring it back to health. If your brain or kidney were in trouble, you'd eat brain or kidney, respectively. If an eye issue were troubling you, you'd be advised to consume the eyeball of an animal in some way, shape, or form. And this wasn't limited to folk remedy, by the way. It was prevailing medical wisdom that doctors learned in the most prestigious medical universities during their training.

The problem with this mode of treatment was that it never worked. Your leg, brain, kidney, eye, or other body part would continue to act up unless you found another mode of healing—not that this was acknowledged. The theory seemed to make so much sense on the surface that it continued to hold credibility straight through from the Middle Ages for hundreds of years. (And believe it or not, it holds credibility in today's nutritional supplement world, where there's still belief that if you ingest a capsule that has brain or liver bile material in it, it will somehow help your own brain or liver.) By the time goiters started to become a widespread problem in the population at the time of the Industrial

Revolution, it was still a theory that doctors carried in their bag of tricks. So one doctor decided to see if offering dried and ground pig thyroid to a goiter patient would bring down the thyroid swelling. For the first time in the history of treating body parts with body parts, it worked. In the 1800s, dehydrated thyroid became a commonplace goiter remedy that you could pick up at the drugstore. No one knew why it brought goiters down, though they were happy to go along with it.

Was it a miracle cure? No. Consuming thyroid worked for these early thyroid patients only because goiters of the time were caused by serious iodine deficiencies (due to industrialized food processing that stripped food of its nutrients), coupled with toxic overload from a polluted environment, and pig thyroid offered them a rich source of iodine to balance their health.

As time went on, widespread iodine deficiency opened the way for the first wave of early, crude Epstein-Barr virus to target the thyroid—though the virus was still so mild that it only took a little dose of iodine, an antiseptic, to kill off the problematic EBV, and the desiccated porcine thyroid provided just that.

Over time, EBV mutated and grew stronger, and people developed bigger problems than iodine-deficiency goiters and not-so-aggressive, low-grade viral goiters—they developed the EBV symptoms we looked at two chapters ago that are mistaken for thyroid symptoms. Still, desiccated thyroid seemed to make a difference in many of these patients. Why? Not because the medication was offering them T4 or T3—it had nothing to do with thyroid hormone replacement. Rather, it was because with desiccated thyroid, the medical establishment had also unknowingly stumbled upon its first steroid compound. The concentrated hormones in the animal thyroid acted as an immunosuppressive, anti-inflammatory drug on some patients—meaning that thyroid swelling would go down, other viral symptoms would abate, and it would *seem* like a person was getting better. In reality, the concoction was causing a shutoff of their immune system response to the EBV.

THE TRUTH ABOUT THYROID HORMONES

Today's thyroid medications are not at all far off from those thyroid drugs of yore. Some of these medications are, in fact, still made of desiccated porcine thyroid. Others are synthetic. Either way, current thyroid medications act as steroids just as those early ones did, though many doctors don't realize this—and no one knows that the steroid effect is why some people may notice a little more energy, mental clarity, and improved sleep when they begin taking thyroid medication. It is partial relief from their low-grade viral infections, and that's all.

Another common reason that some people feel relief or experience weight loss on thyroid medication has nothing to do with the medication itself. As I've said, the overwhelming majority of people who see these improvements

are ones who at the same time they went on a prescription, also changed their diet, went on supplements, and/or got more exercise. It's this removal of EBV's favorite foods coupled with immune-boosting nutrients and lifestyle improvements that changes these people's health for the better. (Taking thyroid medication for years contributes to a sluggish liver and, because the medication is a steroid compound, to underactive adrenals. These factors usually translate to eventual weight gain around the belly and other spots in the body.)

Medical communities are under the mistaken impression that the above improvements are due to thyroid hormone replacement—though again, in truth, it has nothing to do with filling in for hormones that a person's body is having trouble producing or converting. Whether animal or synthetic, the hormones in these medications are not bioidentical to human thyroid hormones, which means they're missing key chemical compounds, which have not yet been discovered, that set human thyroid hormones apart. (Plus, the thyroxine in thyroid medication essentially fakes out the pituitary gland, sending it the message that the thyroid is producing enough of its hormones to suit the body.)

Think of the difference between synthetic thyroxine, desiccated animal thyroxine, and human thyroxine as the difference between feeding a baby factory formula, cow's milk, or breast milk. Enough research has come to light by now that we know that even as close as outside sources may come, breast milk can't be matched. The day will come when research reveals the same about human thyroid hormones. (The only source that can fill in for these hormones comes from within the body—it's the special blend that the adrenals produce in compensation for an underactive thyroid.) When someone has a bad reaction to thyroid medication, which thousands do, it's because her body is so fine-tuned to this difference that it can't tolerate hormones that come from a non-human source.

What we need to keep in mind is that whether a person feels better, worse, or the same on thyroid medication, it is not prescribed for the thyroid itself—it does not heal the thyroid. Many patients are not aware of this. They think that because they went to the doctor and received a prescription to treat their thyroid symptoms, the prescription is treating the problem itself. Meanwhile, the EBV can continue to damage the thyroid (and cause other worsening symptoms), and the thyroid disease can continue to progress. If you take medication for a hypothyroid, you'll still have a hypothyroid, and you'll still have EBV, unless you take the express measures we'll look at in Part III, "Thyroid Resurrection," to get rid of the virus and care for your thyroid.

This explains why you can still be gaining weight, losing hair, feeling fatigued, and generally suffering even after you've gone on medication for thyroid issues. It's a common experience for millions of people: they're diligently taking their medication every day, and even though that medication is causing thyroid test results to indicate normal hormone levels, their thyroids are getting worse over the years, because no one knew to look for the underlying issue and address the real cause.

I've seen people who've had their thyroids removed, and who weren't taking any thyroid medication, feeling great after they got rid of their EBV. I've also seen people who were on thyroid medication, with or without their thyroid, and who hadn't gotten rid of their EBV yet, who felt terrible. If feeling better were all about thyroid hormones, neither of these scenarios would exist—the people missing their thyroids would need thyroid medication to function, and everyone who was on thyroid medication would be restored to health. The reality is that it's all about the thyroid virus, Epstein-Barr. When EBV is present and active, it's going to be a drain on someone's health, regardless of whether she or he is on thyroid medication.

Also, remember those adrenal replica hormones we looked at in Chapter 4, "Your Thyroid's True Purpose"? Because your adrenal glands produce adrenaline blends that replicate thyroid hormones when the thyroid gland is underactive, essentially, your body creates your own medicine. Though close enough to your true thyroid hormones that your body uses them in the same way, they are subtly different enough that blood tests won't pick up these blends as thyroid hormones. As a result, doctors will prescribe thyroid medication not knowing that your endocrine system is producing a dose of its own prescription to fill in for the thyroid's tasks. Where the body really needs help is in immune system support to lower the viral load.

While you're taking the steps in this book to free yourself of EBV, if you'd also like to truly support your thyroid hormones, you can make your own thyroid tonic by following the instructions in Chapter 25, "Thyroid Healing Techniques."

THYROID MEDICATION AND TSH READINGS

It's important to understand the true relationship between TSH readings and thyroid medication—because it's one that's frequently misunderstood.

Here's a common scenario: Your blood test results show a TSH reading of 10.0, which your doctor sees as the start of a hypothyroid issue and so proceeds to offer you medication. After starting on the prescription, you go back for another blood test, and this time your reading is in the 4.0 to 5.0 range. It's easy to think this means your thyroid is being treated.

In fact, all that's happening is that the thyroid hormones in your system from the medication are faking out your pituitary gland, telling it that you're making enough hormones, so that your pituitary will produce less of its thyroid-stimulating hormone. That lower TSH reading gives a false sense of security; your thyroid itself is not getting any relief from the medication. The way your body's truly functioning, that TSH level should still be at 10.0. The medication is merely masking it.

And over time, since the EBV isn't being addressed and it's still highly active inside your thyroid, possibly due to triggers in your life, your thyroid's performance will continue to worsen. That means you'll go back to the doctor after a while on medication, and those TSH levels will have climbed back up again. It's very likely that the doctor will put you on higher and higher dosages of medication. (If you're someone who isn't experiencing many thyroid virus triggers in your life, your thyroid medication dosages may remain steady for a longer period before increasing.) Years down the road, your TSH reading may reach 10.0 again—which means that without the medication obscuring the results, you would really be at a 20.0. The hypothyroidism is not being treated by the medication; it only seems like it is.

This effect of thyroid medication on TSH readings is sort of like slapping a Band-Aid over the poke-hole from a sword's deep, dirty cut. The wound will continue to fester if it's not cared for properly—if someone doesn't say, "Hey, what's this sword wound doing here in the first place?"

Or think of medication's effect on TSH readings like taking the battery out of a smoke detector: while it may put you at ease because the beeping stops, all you've done is disable the alarm system, not put out the fire.

THYROID ATROPHY

It's good to be aware of one side effect of long-term thyroid medication use that's completely unknown to medical research and science: In some people, thyroid medication can train the thyroid to lessen its hormone production, so that the gland slowly atrophies and shrinks over time. Essentially, the medication dumbs down the thyroid.

Just like your muscles need to be used to stay strong, so too does your thyroid need to do its job regularly to stay in shape. You know how when a snowstorm keeps you cooped up indoors, you may feel frustrated at first? If the storm lasts for a while, though, then day by day, you get a little more used to the forced laziness. Staying inside in your pajamas feels more and more comfortable and natural, so that by the time the storm passes, the prospect of digging out and reentering the world seems like too much energy. That's what can happen over time to the thyroid with long-term thyroid medication use. The thyroid loses some of that yearning to produce hormones—its soul is almost hampered—because the medication is telling the pituitary gland that enough T4 and T3 are being produced, so the thyroid doesn't get the TSH signals that keep it in gear.

Not that you should worry. This type of partial thyroid atrophy only happens to some people who've been overmedicated with prescription thyroid hormones for a number of years—it doesn't happen to everyone on thyroid medication. And even as thyroid medication makes less work for the thyroid, the thyroid will defy this and produce *some* thyroid hormone no matter what. Plus, the thyroid's radio-like frequencies that monitor and promote homeostasis will continue to function in the face of atrophy. (Remember, the undiscovered thyroid hormones R5 and R6 that play a role in these frequencies are virtually impossible to deplete.) Still, it's one of those possible side effects you should know about.

As you've seen over and over in this book, your thyroid is resilient. So you should also know that when you start taking the steps to tame EBV and revive your thyroid, it brings the thyroid's intelligence back to life. Your thyroid's highly equipped database is able to override the state of atrophy, and your thyroid returns to functioning the way it's supposed to function.

WHAT TO KNOW ABOUT WEANING OFF THYROID MEDICATION

If lowering or going off of thyroid medication is a decision you've made with your doctor, there are some key points you need to know.

First, when someone consumes a medication such as a thyroid prescription, the liver automatically absorbs and processes it, because the liver is the body's protector from all outside substances. The higher the dosages you've taken, and the longer the time period you've been on them, the more medication your liver has absorbed and is still holding on to. This is not something that's measured at the doctor's office; medical research and science are still ignoring this fact. If you took the liver of someone who'd been on thyroid medication for many years, wrung it out, dehydrated all that medicine you squeezed out, and put it into

capsules. you could fill hundreds of bottles of thyroid medication.

If you've just gone on thyroid medication, your blood tests may not register any difference in your hormone levels at first, because your liver is absorbing most of it so quickly. As a result, your doctor may end up prescribing higher dosages over time, which will likely continue to be soaked up by the liver. At a certain point—it's different for everyone; it could take 10 years—the thyroid medication buildup in the liver can become toxic and burdensome to the organ, and the liver will slowly begin to release the medication back into the bloodstream, sometimes in intermittent spurts, because it's overloaded. When this happens, it will throw off blood tests, making it look to your doctor like you're producing more thyroid hormones than you are—another reason why they are only guess tests and doctors find themselves continually adjusting the protocols for many patients.

Many times, doctors will see your thyroid panels coming back with better levels, and they'll think it's because your thyroid is performing better, when in reality, it's because the liver has reached its fill-up mark and begun releasing medication back into the bloodstream. The medication being released back into your bloodstream is not as active or viable as when you first took it, though. It has only about a 5 percent Band-Aid effect for the body.

And because it backs up into the bloodstream like this—rather than being ingested, breaking down in the stomach, and assimilating through digestion—your body can have an adverse reaction, and you may become intolerant to your medication. This can often result in feeling allergic in some way, where you feel swelling or a racing heart or have difficulty sleeping when you've never had that problem before. When one of these reactions happens, it's common to need to switch from synthetic to compounded natural or vice versa, or even to be forced off of thyroid medication altogether because your body has become so sensitive to it. Even without this overflow effect, thyroid medication taken for an extended period—some people have been on it for over 20 years—can put additional pressure on a liver already made sluggish and stagnant by EBV, which can lead to more weight gain, among other symptoms, over time.

If you've been on thyroid medication for a long time, you may want to talk to your doctor about keeping your dosages lower so your liver can do some detox. Take great care with it, and don't make the decision on your own. Sometimes people decide they want to go cold turkey and stop their thyroid medications all at once. The effect can be overwhelming, with symptoms such as fatigue returning immediately. People often conclude that they need the medication, so they go back on it, feeling that they'll be dependent for life.

Here's what's really going on with those symptoms: First, there's the withdrawal to consider. When someone has been taking a steroid for years, the body goes into shock when those drugs go away abruptly—and the result can be a lot of physical discomfort. Doctors know to wean patients off of other steroids very slowly for this reason, and they should treat thyroid medications no differently.

Secondly, when you stop taking thyroid medication all at once, the liver gets an immediate sense of liberation and releases old thyroid medication it's absorbed over time back into the bloodstream, often very quickly. With all those hormones suddenly in the bloodstream, the body can react adversely, causing the symptoms people mistake as dependence on thyroid medication that are really detox symptoms. For someone who's only been on thyroid medication for three months to a year, the detox may not be that formidable—you may only experience a day or week of feeling a little tired, depending on the dosage you were on. Once you've been taking thyroid medication for over a year, weaning off slowly is especially important so you don't overload your system. This liver detox is ultimately helpful, as it helps unclog t and prevent you from gaining more weight.

When evaluating how long the weaning process should take for patients, doctors should always consider how long someone has been on thyroid medication—it makes a real impact on someone's health and well-being as they lower her or his dosages. If someone has only been on thyroid medication for two to five years, the dosage should be cut by a quarter at a time, stretched out for at least two months. If someone has been on thyroid medication for five to ten years, that weaning process should extend to at least four months. If someone has been on thyroid medication for 10 to 20 years, weaning should take at least six months. And if someone has been on thyroid medication for over 20 years, then the weaning process should take at least a year. It's very important to know that no matter how long patients have been on thyroid medication, their sensitivity needs to be factored in. Someone could already be dealing with neurological fatigue or another neurological symptom or condition caused by EBV, which could amplify that person's reaction when coming down off the medication. If you're the patient looking to lower your dosages, consult with your doctor about what's best for you.

Meanwhile, your thyroid is still producing its own thyroid hormones to some degree, plus your adrenals are producing those hormones that don't register on tests as backup. To give them support, your goal should be to become proactive about knocking EBV out of your system and bringing your thyroid back to health with the tools in this book so the gland can rebalance and produce the hormone levels it's meant to produce. This will support you as the medication leaves your system, so that you have the best chance of feeling great.

LEVELS OF REVELATION

Some advanced medical professionals have caught on to the limits of thyroid testing. They've noticed patients who present with classic hypothyroidism symptoms and whose thyroid panels come back in the normal range. These doctors put the patients on thyroid medication anyway, and sometimes the patients will start to feel better. Finally being taken seriously and heard like this is progress for thyroid patients.

It's far better than the days when a woman would visit the doctor with chronic mystery symptoms and hear that nothing was wrong. "You just need to exercise more," was the advice they'd get. Or, "Find a hobby. You just have too much time on your hands." That's the type of non-diagnosis that can make someone lose all trust in her powers of perception.

The new approach is also more enlightened than when a woman visits the doctor with aches and pains, heart palpitations, weight gain, hair loss, memory loss, and confusion and hears that it's all about hormone imbalance, and that she's going through menopause or perimenopause. This type of diagnosis makes countless women feel old before their time—and as though suffering is a natural part of aging. (It isn't.)

When the thyroid factors into a doctor's evaluation of a patient's chronic health issues, it is progress. When that doctor recognizes that the thyroid may be involved even if tests don't pick up problems, or that a prescription from a compounding pharmacy is better than synthetic, it's all the more enlightened.

And still, these revelations are not there yet. They're advancements for the history books. The truths you've just examined—about how EBV is the real cause of thyroid issues and much more, about what your symptoms really mean, about how thyroid testing works, and about how thyroid medication completely misses and bypasses the underlying cause of your illness— are for your life right now. The revelation that your thyroid is a messenger, not the problem, is the expert-level knowledge you need to ensure a brighter future.

As you move forward with your health, it may be easy to get distracted. New theories will surface, old theories will get revived and recirculated, and you may wonder if the thyroid information you hear about on TV or read about in the latest literature is what you should be listening to instead. Remember this: As long as a thyroid theory puts the blame on you, your body, or triggers alone, it is not correct. As long as a treatment is not going after the underlying virus, it will not solve anything.

To arm you against so much competing and confusing misinformation out there, we'll turn now to the Great Mistakes of chronic illness. By discovering these key blunders that hold back medical advancements, you'll gain new clarity, trust, and freedom—so you can finally heal.

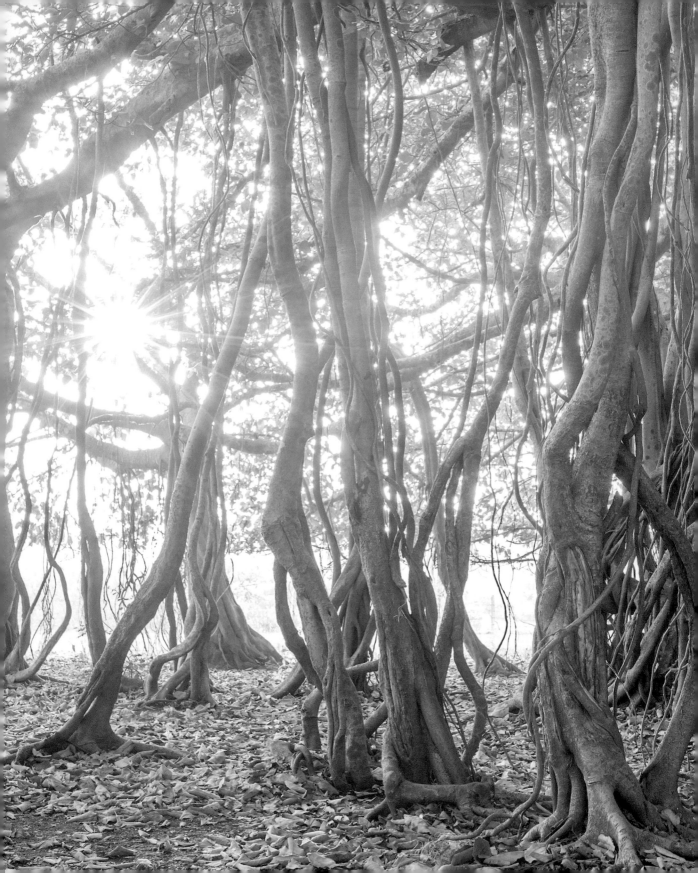

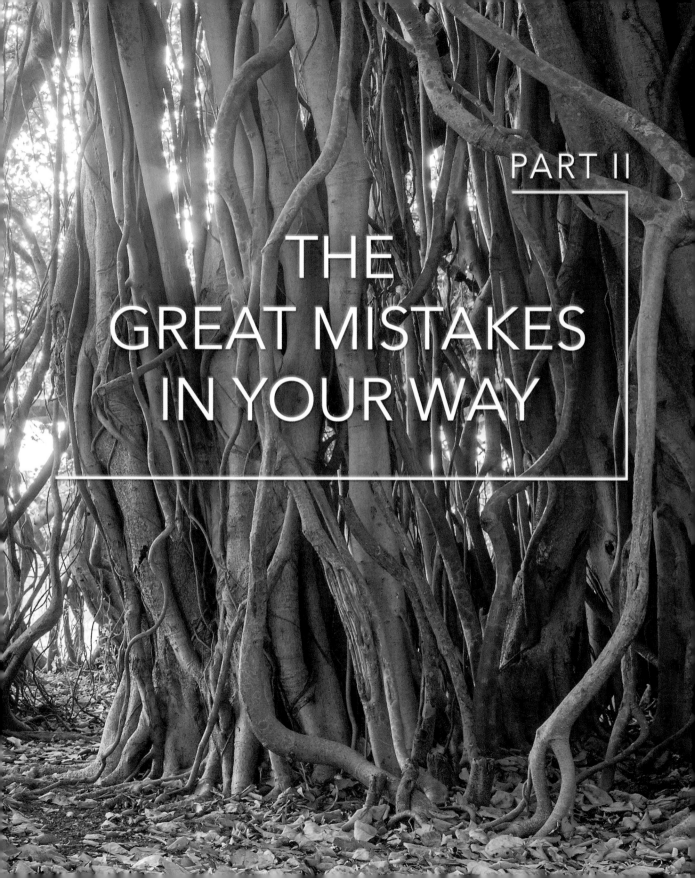

PART II

THE GREAT MISTAKES IN YOUR WAY

CHAPTER 9

A Bridge to Better Health

How do you get from where you are to where you want to be? How do we transport ourselves from this place where we're standing to that place over there, beyond the obstacle? As long as humans have been on the planet, we've been asking these questions—and answering them by building bridges.

It likely started when our ancestors stumbled upon one of nature's bridges—perhaps a fallen tree spanning two river banks—and from there, the idea developed: A gap didn't have to be the end of the path. We could create our own support structures to carry ourselves and each other to new land.

Through the millennia, builders and engineers have developed techniques and technologies to advance bridge building to its place today as one of the highest sciences. We now live in a world where the wonder of these inventions has become commonplace. We walk, bike, or drive over them without necessarily giving them too much consideration. And yet if you stop to think about it, each bridge represents tremendous care. Think about all of the math, physics, design, planning, and then actual construction that go into every one. It takes extraordinary skill to understand and harness the laws of nature and, in the end, create a bridge that's safe and sound for the hundreds, thousands, or millions who will cross it.

What defines bridge building is that it has to be right. In the final product, there's no room for error—because people's lives are at stake. If someone has a high-minded idea for a new bridge design, or a hunch for an improvement on accepted practices, it needs to be tested. Prototypes need to be created, and then more advanced models. Every line must be exact, every angle precise, every calculation quadruple-checked, every material tried and true. All of the elements must be accounted for, and the foundation must be exactly right for that exact terrain.

When it comes to treating chronic illnesses in today's medical communities—to bridging patients' divide between feeling unwell and reaching that promised land of vibrant health—there are no similar calculations to make. Doctors can't measure, weigh, or size up chronic illness; they can't throw specifications into an advanced software system like engineers do and get a visual of what someone's healing path should look like. The funding that will lead medical research and science to the most correct and advanced diagnostics and prescriptions simply isn't there yet. Instead, doctors are left to feel it out. Partly, they rely on those areas of medicine that do get funding and try to apply whatever they can from those tangentially related studies.

Mostly, when it comes to chronic illnesses such as thyroid disease, doctors must rely on theories—theories that I've mentioned in earlier chapters of this book, such as autoimmunity, genetic blame, and metabolism. It probably sounds a little strange to hear them called "theories," because in contemporary medicine, they're treated like fact. And yet, once you investigate them a little more, you come to realize just how many unknowns are supporting them. These are the types of theories that, in bridge building, would have to undergo rigorous testing before they were put into practice. In that testing, they would start to crumble; fissures would form; the weak points would reveal themselves. The experts would realize that, for example, the theory of Hashimoto's thyroiditis as the immune system attacking the thyroid couldn't be offered to people as an answer to explain their suffering, because it wouldn't truly support them. Hearing that your body attacks itself doesn't transport a person to better health, because it's not the truth.

The experts would learn, too, that trying to cover over the cracks with pieces of tape—like pointing to inflammation as cause—couldn't keep those cracks from deepening or the bridge from falling apart.

That's the interesting thing about chronic illness. In this field, the term "expert" is unique. In so many other disciplines—even in other areas of medicine, such as surgery—an expert is someone who understands an issue's underlying cause. An expert surgeon knows how to use a scalpel just right and to stitch up the heart to repair a leaky valve. A legal expert understands the loophole in a law that allowed a criminal to get away with murder. An expert engineer knows, when a bridge falls down, how to acknowledge it, document it, study it, figure out the underlying problem—maybe the wrong grade steel was used—and then address that issue in all future designs.

And yet someone heralded as an expert in thyroid disease or another chronic illness doesn't need to get to the bottom of why those symptoms happen in the first place in order to receive that title of "expert." It's one of the only areas in the trade and professional worlds where it's so gray. As well-meaning as these people are, they're operating off of recycled ideas about what *seems* to cause improvements in *some* patients and going by old theories that have been grandfathered in as acceptable medical advice.

That's why it is time for *you* to become the true thyroid expert in your life. You've already gotten so far by examining the thyroid virus and how it works, the true purpose of your thyroid, the secrets behind what causes the symptoms attributed to thyroid issues and related illnesses, and the truth behind thyroid testing and medication. Now we're going to look at some of the greatest mistakes when it comes to chronic illness. Knowing how to avoid these is one of the most vital elements of building a sound, solid bridge to better health.

GRAVE MISTAKES

Mistakes happen. We all make them. Sometimes we don't even know we're making them—we're just operating on incorrect information from others, and taking their word for it. It's no one's fault, and yet a mistake like this doesn't leave us in any less of a mess.

Say, for example, you drive to the grocery store. Your son's friend is staying with you while his family goes through a tough time, and all he'll eat in his state of distress are cornflakes. This is your one window of time to stock up during a busy day—and when you get to the cereal aisle and look at the shelf, the space for cornflakes is empty. You flag down a clerk. "Excuse me, do you have more of these in the back?" you ask.

"I'll check the storeroom," he says, and hurries away. When he returns, he's empty-handed. "Sorry, we're all out. You'll have to wait until we get our next delivery."

This doesn't sit right. A supermarket out of cornflakes? You ask to speak with the manager. When the clerk brings her to you, you explain your situation. "Are you sure you don't have a single box in the store?"

"Jon already checked the stockroom," the manager says, then catches your eye. "Let's check one more time," she adds. Together, the manager and the clerk disappear. A long while passes as you wait for them to return. Finally, they approach, each holding an armful of cornflake boxes.

"I'm so sorry," the clerk says. "I can't believe I told you that we were out. They were on an unmarked pallet on the opposite side of the room from where they're supposed to be."

"Yes, we apologize," the manager says. "We don't know how this happened, though we won't try to make excuses. I'll walk with you to the registers and tell your checker to give you a discount to make up for our error."

So some people made some honest mistakes. You had to spend a little extra time at the grocery store. And maybe no one was really at fault—maybe the person who usually unpacks deliveries was out sick, and her substitute didn't know the job well enough. In the end, it's no big deal. You caught the mistake and didn't leave empty-handed. Besides, it was just a box of cereal. No one's life was at stake.

The mistakes we make in daily life, even the really bad ones that ripple out to affect others, are still just normal mistakes. They're part of the human experience. Much as they may hurt in the moment, we can try to learn something from them and move on with new wisdom.

A Great Mistake, on the other hand, is no box of cornflakes. It's a mistake that you didn't make, though you have to pay for it—in a big way. A Great Mistake is a grave mistake. It's not any one person's fault, though that doesn't make it any less dangerous. And it's one that's not acknowledged as being a mistake at all.

Have you ever had a joke played on you? It might have felt uncomfortable, annoying, or even disheartening. In the end, you found out it was a joke. You figured out the family member or coworker or friend who had propped the bucket of water at the top of the door so that when you walked through, the bucket tipped, and you got drenched. Maybe it even seemed funny once you understood. Or maybe you didn't ever figure out who did it, which was okay, since at least you knew it had been a practical joke, and it was over.

What if you were tricked or fooled, and you didn't know it was happening? What if for your whole life, there'd been a running joke that no one ever told you about? What if the same joke had been played on your parents, and they never knew, either? What if it had been played on your grandparents, too, and your great-grandparents and great-great-grandparents and great-great-great-grandparents? That wouldn't be a funny joke at all, though at least it had been put to rest for those ancestors who had passed.

What if the joke were still being played, though—on your children and on your children's children? That wouldn't be a joke anymore. It would be unthinkable. It would be a Great Mistake.

We're taught in today's society that we always have a choice in life. No matter what, we hear, we have the power to choose our direction. Well, a joke that you're never let in on takes away that freedom of choice. A running gag that's silently held you back in life, and that's now holding back your children, takes away your right to find something better—because you don't even know these limits are in place.

Back before the women's suffrage movement in the U.S., when women weren't allowed to vote, it was acknowledged in many circles that it was wrong. What allowed it to change eventually was that it wasn't a secret rule. It was out in the open that law prohibited women from voting. Women and their supporters knew that this wasn't how it should be, and so they had the choice to take a stand and fight for the right for women to cast their own ballots.

Because the Great Mistakes are hidden in plain sight, you don't get that same choice. You don't know what opportunities you're missing out on—unless you discover the truth.

THE GREAT MISTAKES OF CHRONIC ILLNESS

Chronic illness has reached such an epidemic level that I call it an *epic-demic*. And with the Great Mistakes of chronic illness, the stakes are just as high as they were for women's suffrage. Millions of people are living limited lives, held back from experiencing a basic human right—in this case, the right to good health—though it's been in secret. We aren't being told that these are Great Mistakes holding back millions of people, so nobody knows to stand up against them. They are so ingrained that they seem like the facts of life. We trust them, just as we trust that if a road leads to a bridge, it's safe to drive over. If there are no orange cones or detour signs, we believe that the authorities have everything in order, and we should follow where others have gone before us.

And yet the truth is that the medical theories, trends, and misconceptions that make up the Great Mistakes are, indeed, mistakes. Some of them have been holding us back for generations and will continue to hold back future generations unless they're stopped. Many of them started as genuine efforts to help people, or to impress colleagues with high-level reasoning, and then, like jokes gone bad or runaway trains, they gained momentum. Now everyone has gotten on these trend trains, and they're going so fast that their sheer speed seems like confirmation that they're on the right track. No one realizes that the trains' conductors and engineers long ago lost control, and that the trains are now barreling along on their own.

Some of these mistakes, like the belief that you created your illness, are new enough that the emergency brake can still be used, and we can bring the train to a stop. Others, like the autoimmune theory, are going at such a dangerous velocity that the only way to save yourself is to jump from the escape hatch to the getaway car before that train derails. When you discover the truth about the Great Mistakes, you get the safety mechanisms you need to protect yourself and the ones you love, and you get back the freedom that you didn't even know you lost.

The nine Great Mistakes of chronic illness which we'll delve into one by one as we move through Part II, are:

- Autoimmune Confusion
- Mystery Illness Misconception
- Labels as Answers
- Inflammation as Cause

- Metabolism Myth
- Gene Blame Game
- Ignoring the Unforgiving Four
- It's All in Your Head
- You Created Your Illness

These are mistakes that cause widespread suffering; take away your choice, freedom, and rights; and leave you feeling like you're to blame. These are mistakes that are not owned up to and acknowledged, where you don't get to call in the manager and ask her to go back and double-check for you. After applying a Great Mistake to you, no one returns later admitting they'd been looking in the wrong place for an answer. Nor are the Great Mistakes recalled, as they should be, like a batch of ground beef found to be contaminated with *E. coli.* "We're sorry," the announcement would go, "these ideas are not safe to consume. Return them for a full refund of your mental health."

Have you ever been sharing the story of your thyroid woes with others, and that look comes into their eyes that means they're not quite with you anymore? Whether it's the first time you've told your story to them or the umpteenth update, there's a subtle or not-so-subtle skepticism that can creep into the mind of someone who's trying to bear witness to a friend, patient, or loved one dealing with chronic illness. It's skepticism that's borne out of the Great Mistakes clouding their thoughts. *Why hasn't this person gotten better with so many answers available to them?* these people wonder. And instead of the next thought being, *There must be something wrong with the information,* they think, *There must be something wrong with this person.* This kind of thinking can start to creep into your own mind with any symptom or condition you're dealing with, and it can be so destructive.

You already know—on some level, however deeply you've had to bury this knowing—that you're not doing anything wrong, and that the Great Mistakes aren't answers. You've already lived through several if not all of them. If they were answers, you wouldn't still be searching for the path to health.

There are no fingers to point in the misguided theories of chronic illness. As I said, we all make mistakes. And we've all had experiences of unknowingly carrying out mistakes that were not our own. The true mark of progress is not how few wrong turns we make; it's how deftly we correct course when we learn we've been going in the wrong direction.

In order to correct course, we really need to know what went wrong. We need to be able to point to the map and say, "See? This is how far away we are from where we meant to go. These are the spots where we misread the road signs." Otherwise, how do we find the right path?

Mostly, the Great Mistakes have been the result of medical denial. And like all denial, this gets in the way of progress. It upholds an illusion of functionality—when meanwhile, things are falling apart. People dealing with the reality of chronic illness feel disposable, crumpled up and thrown away like dirty tissues. It may be uncomfortable to face this reality—that's okay. It is far, far better to feel some discomfort about the truth than to repeat these mistakes for the next 50 years, which is what's bound to happen unless these truths surface.

If you need another reference point for the Great Mistakes, just think of the Great Lakes, which were so polluted by the 1960s that Lake Erie was pronounced to be "dying." This was another tragedy caused by human error. Eventually, environmentalists rallied around the cause, legislation was passed, steps were taken to limit fertilizer runoff and pollutants, and life returned to the lake. In recent years, dead zones have been reported again, and people are once more calling for pollution control.[2]

We can use this story as a touchstone for the Great Mistakes to come. Just as the citizens of the Lake Erie watershed once made tremendous progress in bringing the lake back to life, so too can medical communities change their direction when it comes to how they view chronic conditions such as thyroid illness—if enough people rally around the cause. Course-correcting for human error takes constant vigilance. We can't let appearance of improvement lull us into complacency. Just as it still takes close observation and advocacy for the truth to keep the lake's best interest in the public eye, we can all keep our eye out for one another to ensure that progress remains forward-moving.

OUT OF ANTIQUITY

To get perspective on today's Great Mistakes of chronic illness, we must keep in mind that one day, we'll look back at the present as a moment in history. Science's hallmark is that its study develops over time to allow for a deeper, richer, truer understanding of our world. New experiments improve upon old ones; clear insights replace mistaken hypotheses; "advancements" that went in the wrong direction for the wrong reasons get reeled back in and redirected. So what may seem like the forefront of rational thought today could one day be considered out-of-date as new facts come to light. This is the perspective we must bring to analyzing modern-day medical theories: some will stand the test of time; others won't.

Take, for example, the time when tonsillectomies first drew favor. Many children began presenting with tonsillitis, and the prevailing

wisdom became that the tonsils should be removed. It became such dominant thinking that no one even thought to question whether the cause of tonsillitis in the first place could be addressed instead. The focus on the medical advancement of the tonsillectomy procedure completely buried the mystery of this widespread tonsillitis. Once tonsillectomies became commonplace, someone in medical school wouldn't be encouraged to probe the problem anymore, because it had become "been there, done that." Remove the tonsils, the thinking went, and remove the problem. Why spend any more time thinking about it?

Medical communities now recognize that the tonsils are tied into the immune system, and so removing them isn't the best first option when they're infected. Now antibiotics have become the favored first line of defense. This is problematic, because while cofactor bacteria can further inflame the tonsils, bacteria are not the underlying cause of tonsillitis; EBV is. This whole time, it's been juvenile Epstein-Barr virus causing inflamed tonsils. In children, EBV is very difficult to diagnose, because it often doesn't raise red flags that testing can detect in the bloodstream. Meanwhile, the lymphatic area where the tonsils reside can become infected as they try to fight off the virus, causing the mystery tonsil infection. It's another instance of hidden mononucleosis—and the history of medical research and science being mistaken about how to solve a problem.

Or consider the era when breastfeeding was discouraged. Several decades ago, breastfeeding was considered inferior to the brand-new, scientifically created baby formulas that were hitting the market. Women were told to stop breastfeeding, because science knew better than the human body. (For perspective, this happened to coincide with the time when cars didn't have headrests to prevent whiplash and seat belts only went across the lap—and yet cars were considered advanced.) Families respected this advice and regarded formula as God . . . until the research surfaced years later that breast milk has untold value. The paradigm started to shift as more and more people came to realize that the human body *can* be trusted, and that science is in fact the one lagging behind—though unfortunately this realization has stayed limited to this one area.

So you get the idea about how one day, we'll look back on today's medical approach to thyroid disease and other chronic illnesses from a whole new vantage point: as antiquity. In contemporary conventional medicine, there are three main treatments for a chronic issue:

steroids (including hormone treatments and immunosuppressants), antibiotics, and procedures to remove the perceived problem. You might have received all three. And if one or all of them didn't make you feel better, it's very likely you got the message that you are the problem. This will, one day, change. The development and practice of medicine will evolve.

Because the truth is, you're not the problem, and you didn't do anything wrong. The information to come about the Great Mistakes will show you what *has* been wrong all along—what type of thinking to avoid, and what pitfalls to side-step. They will show you that you can trust yourself again, and that you can use that trust to get yourself from where you are with your health to where you want to be.

CHAPTER 10

Great Mistake 1: Autoimmune Confusion

Even at its most basic, the autoimmune theory is misguided. That's right—the term *auto-immune* itself is a huge mistake. *Auto-* comes from the Greek for "self," so the word is saying that your immune system goes after you—your own self! That makes *autoimmune* merely a tag that puts the blame on you and your body. It's a misnomer that means we can't even talk about the truth of autoimmune disease without perpetuating the misunderstanding. A more fitting term would be *viral-immune*, because the immune system is going after invaders. *Autoimmune* is not just a mistaken fixation of the conventional medical world. Alternative, functional, and integrative circles have also adopted this misconception.

Why does this theory exist? Because by the 1950s, the medical world became frustrated with not having an explanation for why conditions such as Hashimoto's thyroiditis, Graves' disease, lupus, RA, Crohn's disease, celiac disease, ulcerative colitis, and MS were leaving people ailing or even crippled. Close observation of some patients' blood work revealed the presence of antibodies. An exhausting guessing game began, and the theory that best protects

the medical establishment took off: "It must be the body becoming confused and attacking itself." Suddenly, it turned into whisper-down-the-lane on a global scale—except instead of the message becoming garbled along the way, it became glorified and amplified, drowning out the undiscovered truth.

Attempting to explain autoimmune issues was an honest effort at trying to give people answers, except unlike the cornflake story in the last chapter, no manager intervened to say, "Let's check one more time," and then, "Turns out we were looking in the wrong place." Instead, the message that autoimmune disease is the body attacking itself became law.

Now the autoimmune theory is becoming a monster tsunami, or a blizzard blinding everyone to the truth. It's the train barreling down the tracks at a dangerous speed, out of control.

It's time to step back and reevaluate. It's time to band together and voice the truth: The theory that autoimmune disease is the body attacking itself is incorrect. *The body does not attack itself.* It attacks pathogens. (The scientific tests to fully detect those pathogens that are causing trouble simply haven't been invented yet.) Without accepting this truth, the study of autoimmune disease will not move forward in the right direction. The field will remain in a state of confusion, at the expense of all those who suffer with these debilitating symptoms. This is no half hour wasted searching for cornflakes; the consequences of not admitting this mistake will be devastating. It can ruin lives—it already has, and it will continue to into the future.

You'll hear from some sources that autoimmune responses happen when your body is defending itself against a trigger (such as a pathogen or gluten) and becomes confused in the process, unable to tell the difference between a foreign presence and your own body tissue. As we looked at in the triggers chapter, this is *not* how triggers work. Any antibody activity is because those antibodies are going after the virus, not your own body. Remember, your body loves you unconditionally.

It's also important to keep in mind that while science has advanced in its understanding of many aspects of physical function, the thyroid gland remains largely a mystery. There isn't much more medical insight into the thyroid today than there was 100 years ago, which makes it that much easier for medical communities to label thyroid conditions as autoimmune—because it's difficult to assess what's wrong with an organ or gland if the organ or gland itself is a mystery, and "autoimmune" is a convenient tag for, "We don't know what's wrong with you, so it must be your fault."

It's not doctors' fault, either, that any of this is the case. Doctors and other practitioners are heroes who selflessly devote their lives to helping others. They simply haven't yet been handed the best diagnostic tools or framework to determine what's truly going on with their patients who suffer from Hashimoto's, Graves', and other autoimmune diseases.

Medical science is not doomed to misunderstanding autoimmune disease forever. Researchers can still make profound progress in this area and discover the secrets we're looking at in this book—if and only if they first scrap the erroneous theory behind autoimmune and begin again with a new foundation. Once medical science finally taps into the underlying truth about autoimmunity, the study and treatment of thyroid disease and other chronic illnesses will finally be able to advance.

Only then will medical research uncover that the body never attacks itself; it solely goes after pathogens. Antibodies are signs that there's a virus (or other antigen) in the body that the immune system is putting all its energy into fighting off. This process of a pathogen invading cells creates the inflammation. Your body works to fight off that pathogen. One day, medical science will take into account that by the time a virus has started to cause chronic illness in a patient, it has usually burrowed so deep into that person's organs that the virus doesn't show up on traditional blood tests—so it appears to be a bodily malfunction. Hopefully on the sooner side, though most likely far down the road, new tests will develop to find the virus where it's hiding.

Let's remember that medical science is already advancing in so many areas. It has made leaps and bounds in organ transplants, microscopic surgery, and the like—areas that haven't been stymied by denial, areas where a diagnosis can be made and the next steps are clear. It's like when you take your car into the shop, and the mechanic can tell from observation or computer diagnostics what's wrong. If the brakes are worn out, they can get replaced. If the starter is loose, the bolts can be tightened. When the car trouble is outside the realm of easily detectable problems, though, fixing it requires troubleshooting. This can turn into a long guessing game. Unless your mechanic is really invested in getting to the bottom of it, the problem can slip through the cracks at the auto shop, and you'll be back on the road again, still hearing that strange noise.

Has the autoimmune label made you feel like you've slipped through the cracks of the health-care world? Have you visited specialist after specialist, tried every alternative therapy, and felt like you were a disappointment when you couldn't tell your practitioners you'd felt any improvement with their troubleshooting? Did it feel at a certain point like people gave up on you? If so, you're not alone.

So many Hashimoto's and Graves' patients are told that the immune system mysteriously produces antibodies that target and damage the thyroid gland as though it were a foreign presence. This hypothesis will not hold up over time, because it's not the real answer.

If I went to a doctor already feeling low because I had extreme fatigue, a swollen throat, and temperature sensitivity, and that doctor told me it was a result of my body becoming confused and mistaking healthy cells for intrusive ones, I would be beside myself wondering what I did wrong to make my body go haywire. I would feel defective, broken, faulty, inadequate. "Autoimmune" is one of the greatest mistakes of all time. The diagnostic framework points blame in the wrong direction. It makes people think their bodies are betraying them. Once they

stop trusting their bodies, they lose faith that they can heal.

Now, what if you went to the doctor with those symptoms I described, and your doctor answered, "Your body is putting up an amazing fight against a virus, which has been in your system for years undetected and has now reached an advanced stage. That inflammation in your throat is an indication that your body is warding off viral cells that are trying to cause damage to your thyroid. Your fatigue and tendency to run cold come from viral neurotoxins taking a toll on your nerves. I know those symptoms are difficult to deal with. Take heart that they're signs your body is helping you, because remember: Our bodies work for us. They protect us. They love us unconditionally.

"Since this is a viral issue, let's address it with natural means that will kill off that virus. Let's put you on an antiviral eating plan with lots of healing foods, herbs, and supplements to destroy the pathogen and nourish your nerves and thyroid tissue. In the meantime, if you're suffering greatly with body pain, we can always temporarily put you on an immunosuppressive drug or steroid to get you by until your healing protocol has you feeling better."

Wouldn't hearing this make a tremendous difference in how you saw your illness, and in your outlook for recovery? It would have the added benefit of being God's honest truth— and the real way to cut through the autoimmune confusion.

CHAPTER 11

Great Mistake 2: Mystery Illness Misconception

The great mistake of mystery illness is so dire that I wrote my entire first book about it. Here's the short version: Chronic illness is a widespread mystery. Don't be fooled by the popular belief that "mystery illness" is a term that merely applies to rare instances where a few kids in a remote town come down with unexplained rash and fever.

A mystery illness is any ailment that leaves anyone perplexed for any reason. It doesn't matter if that ailment is named or unnamed. Hypothyroidism, Hashimoto's, Graves', hyperthyroidism, and thyroid nodules, cysts, and tumors remain just as enigmatic to modern medicine as inexplicable paralysis that has no label. If you can't visit a practitioner's office and walk away with reasonable answers and a plan that eventually heals you (and doesn't just manage your symptoms), the illness is a medical mystery.

Between symptoms and diseases, there are a minimum of 5,000 health issues that are still a mystery to medical science today. Acting as though migraines, depression, Lyme disease, RA, fatigue, *Candida*, hot flashes, heart palpitations, diabetes, and so many other problems aren't baffling to experts is like ignoring the iceberg that the *Titanic*'s about to strike. This holds true for all the Great Mistakes; pretending they aren't there doesn't make them less of a hazard.

People wonder why so much of the population is sick, and why the cures aren't available yet. It's not because doctors are doing anything wrong. Doctors are some of the smartest, most honest people around—that's what led them to enter the health field in the first place. The trouble is that they're stuck dealing with a system that's broken and can be dishonest, one that's in denial, one that can't always admit when it doesn't have all the answers for fear this unknowing will damage its credibility. It is massively misguided to act as though chronic illnesses such as autoimmune disease are not mysteries to the world at large. It prevents patients from asking for answers, researchers from pursuing them and getting funding, and practitioners from being open to the information they need to help more people.

In reality, the fix here would be to acknowledge how much of human health is still a mystery to science—that's what will bring the awareness and drive to find answers. Only by acknowledging the truth can we redirect course.

CHAPTER 12

Great Mistake 3: Labels as Answers

Don't even get me started on labels. So many of the names that medical science gives to chronic illnesses throw people off the path of finding real answers. As we looked at, one of the biggest is "autoimmune"—the name itself is wrong. When you take it the next step and give labels to all the different autoimmune diseases, the situation gets even more out of hand.

Being labeled with "Hashimoto's," "Graves'," "lupus," "rheumatoid arthritis," and so on can have a positive side. Putting a name with your symptoms can help you feel validated and can also help if your illness is very advanced and you need to be categorized as disabled to get support. When you're struggling with autoimmune disease or another chronic illness, every little bit of recognition helps.

The problem is when we look at labels as answers—as we so often do. Labels make us docile. Telling a patient she or he has Addison's disease, sarcoidosis, psoriasis, alopecia, Castleman disease, endometriosis, Guillain-Barré syndrome, inflammatory bowel disease, Sjögren's syndrome, or the like makes it seem like that's that, and it's all understood. The patient doesn't feel empowered to keep asking, "Why?" and

"What's the underlying cause?" and "Do the studies on this illness seem conclusive?"—to stand up for her or his health rights.

You know how in high school, labels kept everyone from looking beneath the surface? How once someone was deemed to be a burnout, Deadhead, hipster, Goth, freak, teacher's pet, loser, poser, liar, faker, phony, cheater, hypochondriac, sissy, wimp, prep, nerd, jock, techie, slut, emo, klepto, stoner, hippie, or so on, she or he was pigeonholed for the next four years? It didn't matter if you were only playing baseball because your dad was pressuring you to go after sports scholarship money, and in your spare time, you wrote poetry and helped out on archaeological digs. Once people labeled you as a dumb jock, they were finished exploring your personality. It became easy to feel like maybe you really were the person they saw you as, and not the one you felt like inside.

Don't let yourself be pigeonholed by a diagnosis as though this were still high school. First of all, misdiagnosis is rampant in chronic illness. Because these conditions are a mystery and often outside the scope of testing, it often comes down to a practitioner's observation to give you a name for your suffering. That name can be a mistake.

Secondly, the names behind diagnoses don't hold much weight. After all, what's "Hashimoto's thyroiditis" telling us? That a man by the name of Hashimoto observed some thyroids that were inflamed. (That's all –itis means: inflammation.) He made those observations in the early 1900s, by the way, by feeling inflamed thyroids with his hands, a practice that was actually very helpful for getting in touch with the patient's symptoms and has now fallen out of favor. One hundred years later, we are still in the Dark Ages when it comes to how to alleviate the underlying cause of Hashimoto's—unless you've read the detailed information in this book or in the "Hypothyroidism and Hashimoto's Thyroiditis" chapter of *Medical Medium*. That's where the explanation was revealed for the first time.

If you've been given a label for your chronic health struggles and that label makes you feel any level of despair, take heart that you haven't been handed the full reason for your suffering. When you're given the real reason for why you're not feeling your best—not just a name for your limitations—hopelessness disappears, because knowing what's wrong is the first step in healing.

CHAPTER 13

Great Mistake 4: Inflammation as Cause

"Inflammation" is its own label that gets thrown around too liberally. You see inflammation deemed to be the cause of everything from cancer to obesity to heart disease, and it's a huge topic in thyroid illness and autoimmune disease. Everywhere you turn, supplements and health foods are being advertised as anti-inflammatory. It's become a catchall word that we no longer question.

The mistake is not in observing inflammation or in trying to alleviate it. The mistake is in thinking that "inflammation" is an answer. It's not. It's a lazy term, an easy out. Inflammation is not spontaneous, nor is it a lone operator. Rather, it's an indicator. What needs our attention are the true underlying causes behind the inflammation—causes that include the many varieties and strains of Epstein-Barr, shingles, HHV-6, other undiscovered strains such as HHV-10 and HHV-12, and antibiotic-resistant bacteria such as *Streptococcus* and *H. pylori*. As we looked at in Chapter 5, "Your Symptoms and Conditions—Explained," inflammation occurs as a result of invasion and/or injury, and these pathogens can cause both.

Instead, so-called inflammatory foods get the blame. Grains are a major example. Especially in the alternative health community, grains are pegged as causing inflammation and even creating autoimmune disease itself. The buzzword is *mycotoxins* (tiny fungi that can infect grain crops), and it's the explanation many sources use for why grains are problematic. The problem with this logic is that plenty of people eat grains and feel fine. How to explain the 90-year-olds who have spent their lives eating grains and processed foods and have never had a health complaint? What's really going on is that those with autoimmune disease have viruses in their bodies, and those bugs feed on the grains and fungi, resulting in inflammation. So someone who's perfectly pathogen-free won't react to grains, because the grains don't set off a viral feeding frenzy. Someone with Hashimoto's, Sjögren's, scleroderma, MS, or RA, though, will likely feel foggy-headed and fatigued from eating something like bread or bagels.

Inflammation is a good start in acknowledging the suffering that people with chronic illness endure. It's a necessary step, just like before the initial pollution in Lake Erie could be addressed, someone had to first point to the algal bloom. The next step in the path to cleaning up Lake Erie was to question what the algae was communicating, to figure out what was really going on beneath the surface.

Instead, inflammation itself remains the medical focus. It used to be that every doctor would have a different opinion about what label to give a patient's observed inflammation. Now both conventional and alternative medical research and science are stuck in a cycle of testing for levels of inflammation in the body and still playing a guessing game about what to call it. Lupus and psoriatic arthritis are prime examples.

You need to know that tests such as erythrocyte sedimentation rate (ESR), C-reactive protein (CRP), and plasma viscosity (PV), immunoglobulin A (IgA), immunoglobulin G (IgG), and antinuclear antibodies (ANA) are nowhere near conclusive—and that there is monetary gain to be had for the labs that advertise increasingly "advanced" inflammation testing. The tests aren't actually able to determine what's wrong with a person. Rather, the labs come up with charts that arbitrarily match different illness names to the different levels of inflammation. This means that merely because your inflammation markers are at a certain level, you could be diagnosed with Lyme disease versus RA. They are, like thyroid tests, merely guess tests, and they use your inflammation against you to put you in a box and give you a label—instead of interpreting your inflammation to help you so you can heal.

Lately, the charts that labs use to analyze blood test results have started to incorporate pathogen names next to those different levels of inflammation. They do not test for the pathogens themselves, even though they represent that they do, nor have they identified the true pathogens that correspond with different chronic inflammatory illnesses. The blood lab doesn't tell your doctor it hasn't tested for a pathogen itself, though the doctor assumes it has, and this leads the patient to believe a given pathogen was systematically tested for and located. There's a disconnected relationship between the doctor and the blood lab.

This is why you can get tested for Lyme disease and hear that your results are borderline—because the inflammation markers in your blood land on the fringes of a zone where they've listed one or more trendy bacteria that modern medicine mistakenly believes cause Lyme disease. (As I revealed in my first book, it's not bacteria that cause Lyme disease; Lyme disease is viral. If this is winding you up right now, please read the Lyme chapter in *Medical Medium* before you get too upset.) Even putting bacterium versus virus aside, if you have any pathogen in your system, no matter what it is, it's either there or it isn't. Yes, as we established in Chapter 7, "Thyroid Guess Tests," testing still leaves a lot of room for error, so a pathogen in someone's system may not be detected. If it can be detected, though, there's no in-between. It's not possible that you could be borderline. You either see it or you don't. This means that the Lyme test and others like it that go by inflammation markers are completely unstable.

I mention Lyme because it's showing us where this inflammation craze is headed for other chronic illnesses. Inflammation will get all the attention in coming years and obscure the truth that no one's telling you why you're inflamed in the first place. Lyme is such a trendy diagnosis that if a patient has the slightest bit of mystery inflammation caused by any pathogen at all, she or he is likely to get a Lyme diagnosis before the test results have even come back from the lab. Eventually, genes will get the blame for Lyme disease, and countless people will be left feeling like their very essence—their DNA—is to blame for their suffering.

It's worth noting that almost everybody who has Lyme disease has a thyroid problem, whether it's been discovered yet or not. That's because, as I said, Lyme is viral. Usually, someone with Lyme has multiple viruses at once, and one of those is almost always EBV, which if it's far enough along to cause Lyme symptoms, has also interfered with thyroid function. This means that it's common to get multiple diagnoses (e.g., Hashimoto's, hypothyroidism, Lyme) when in reality, there's only one thing wrong—viral

infection—rather than multiple different source problems. Going on an antiviral protocol helps alleviate all of it.

When you know that mystery inflammation is not your body destroying itself and creating your illness—that in fact, this inflammation is a sign that an invader is present, and your body is going after that invader—your whole outlook on your health can change. Rather than pointing to your body as the problem, you can stand confident in the knowledge that there's a greater truth to be discovered about what's causing your chronic symptoms. Stay aware of this Great Mistake, and you'll be able to protect yourself and your family from the dangers of distraction.

CHAPTER 14

Great Mistake 5: Metabolism Myth

The term *metabolism* is far outdated. While it may seem like a concept that's well understood by modern science, with massive volumes of data to back it up, the truth is that *metabolism* refers only to the long-ago discovery that the body is a living organism that assimilates food and uses it for energy. In the several hundred years since this revelation occurred, medicine has not yet cracked the code about why people struggle with their weight. And still, the term is offered up as an answer and explanation—one more label that makes people feel like who they are at their core is to blame for their health issues.

It's a myth that a "slow metabolism" is responsible for someone's difficulty losing weight. This concept is like a vintage car that in its day was the height of beauty and sophistication, a car that got you around for years. Over time, though, it got old. It became outdated. Someone parked it in the backyard, where it started to get rusty. The floorboards rotted, the engine seized up, it became a health hazard as it leaked oil and leached metals into the grass. Only no one could let it go. It was too familiar, held too much sentimental value.

The concept of metabolism has been grandfathered into modern medicine from a time when early medical schools were funded and contracted to teach theories like this one. (Many of the other Great Mistakes have been perpetuated for the same reason.) Metabolism is a convenient idea to hold on to, because it *seems* to offer patients an explanation for their suffering. Theories like this take on a life of their own—a life so large and dominant that it makes doubters seem like fools for questioning them. If you stop to think about it, though, the metabolism theory is not very scientific, and it has a pretty obvious hole: You can't measure metabolism in a definitive way. Isn't science all about objective measurement? If all we have are crude tests that inaccurately estimate how many calories a person burns (it is impossible to truly measure someone's calorie burn), how can we say with any authority that metabolism is the driving force of mystery weight issues?

If solving mystery weight problems were really about eating fewer calories than you burn or measuring your heartbeats per minute, people's problems would already be solved. That advice is so prevalent—everyone's heard it—and so clear-cut that everyone with a weight issue would have followed it and found relief by now. Instead, many people follow calorie-counting advice, don't get results, or find the weight comes right back, and get labeled as lazy or told they're not doing it right.

So if weight problems aren't just about balancing the calories you consume with the calories you expend, what are they about? In some cases, it has to do with the pituitary gland, the kidney, intestinal issues, or even the heart. An overwhelming amount of the time, weight problems are about the liver and the lymphatic system. When someone is overloaded with toxins in their environment, a diet too high in fat or full of unproductive foods, or—as we looked at in Chapter 5—dealing with a viral issue such as EBV, the liver and lymphatic system become overburdened. They can't detox like they're meant to, and when your body can't detox, then like unwanted houseguests, those toxins stick around, clogging up the works. As a protection mechanism, your body retains fluids to keep the toxins suspended, and the resulting edema translates to weight gain. Instead of investigating and uncovering all this, the easy out that gets no one anywhere is to tell someone it's a slow metabolism.

Often, thyroid problems are thought to be the underlying reason for chronic weight issues. Maybe you've been told that your hypothyroidism is to blame for that stubborn weight you can't lose, because your underactive thyroid is failing to produce enough metabolism-boosting hormones to keep your weight in check. Don't let this mistaken theory distract you. It's simply another misconception based on the myth that the speed of the metabolism determines someone's ability to control her or his weight. There is literally no such thing as a slow metabolism—so saying that the thyroid is to blame for a slow

metabolism just makes the theory more wrong. It's just one more scapegoat—what I call an *escape-goat*—for undiscovered health issues like EBV.

The reason weight problems often coincide with thyroid problems is because EBV can cause both—separately. It's not a game of dominos, with EBV knocking into the thyroid, which in turn throws weight off balance. Instead, it's a game of ambush, with EBV advancing to multiple locations in the body, causing problems directly in multiple ways.

When people go on thyroid medication, their weight problems don't go away. That's because thyroid hormones don't regulate weight. In fact, people often gain weight on thyroid medication, because the liver has to absorb the excess thyroxine from the medication, burdening the organ further. As we looked at in Chapter 8, "Thyroid Medication," the overwhelming majority of people who lose weight on thyroid medication do so because they've changed their diet, exercise, and/or supplementation regimen at the same time. The weight loss isn't because of the thyroid hormones revving up the metabolism.

While the thyroid plays a starring role in maintaining the body's homeostasis, and homeostasis is key to your body reaching a balanced weight, the thyroid and the rest of the endocrine system continue to play that role even when the gland is compromised. Finding homeostasis—coming back home in your body—is not about focusing on the thyroid. It's all about detoxing. If you have EBV, it's about getting the virus and its waste matter out of your system and cleansing the toxins and foods that fuel it using the techniques in Part III, "Thyroid Resurrection." These techniques are also excellent for cleansing toxins and reorienting your diet to be more liver- and lymphatic-friendly even if you don't have EBV. They're not about retreating for a month to do a juice cleanse—they're about finding ways to incorporate detoxing into your daily, active life. And they're a world apart from those multivitamins you'll see advertised to support the metabolism. Those ads should say, "This pill will help you find Sasquatch," for how much basis in reality their claims hold.

It's important to note that before and after cleansing toxins, your metabolism remains the same. Whether your liver and lymphatic system are sluggish or in top working order, and whether your thyroid is underactive, overactive, or functioning normally, your metabolism continues on autopilot. That's because when we talk about metabolism, all we're really saying is that we're living, breathing human beings with moving body systems. Those who say otherwise—those who say that metabolism explains someone's hunger and weight—don't understand the true causes of chronic symptoms and illness. And that's okay. It's no one's fault but the old road maps of the past.

I understand that metabolism may be difficult to accept as a Great Mistake, because it's such a part of our everyday language. That ordinariness, though, is part of what makes it so detrimental—the concept is so accepted, no one feels it can even be questioned. With "metabolism" as part of everybody's vocabulary, it's that much more okay to blame someone for her symptoms, which makes it that much more okay for research to stop looking for the real answers. When you see the metabolism theory for what it is, though, you make a difference in the world. You let go of this heavy baggage, and it frees you up to help someone else see that her weight struggles are not her fault.

CHAPTER 15

Great Mistake 6: Gene Blame Game

If you've dealt with chronic symptoms or conditions like the ones we've looked at in this book, you've probably had the belief drilled into you that your body has let you down—which might well have caused you to feel like you committed some cosmic wrong to deserve this punishment. Blaming chronic illness on your genes (as recent theories do) is yet one more way of reinforcing this sense of guilt.

The movement afoot to blame chronic illness on genetics is a classic example of taking a scientific truth, like the fact that we all have DNA and that it plays a profound role in our lives, and then spinning it. Of course genes are real, and we witness their evidence every day in a father's and son's same smile, in the new baby who got his grandmother's nose, and in the voice answering the telephone that you could swear is your sister and turns out to be your niece.

We can't be fooled into thinking genes mean *everything*. They don't determine our entire lives. Our bodies are geared to be well, and outside factors are what create the slew of chronic issues that hold back so many people. After all, chronic illness has quadrupled in the population over the last 30 years. If we follow the genetic logic, wouldn't that mean that genes have gone bad over the past three decades? That doesn't add up.

When you're led to believe that you're suffering because your genes are mutated, distorted, bad, or dysfunctional, it creates a powerful message inside the consciousness of your being that can hold back your healing. If you're told that your illness is a fundamental part of you, how are you supposed to have hope for feeling better?

Whether your challenge is hypothyroidism, hyperthyroidism, Hashimoto's, Graves', thyroid nodules, cysts, tumors, or another chronic issue, know that your condition is not a judgment on your family line, or who you are as a person, nor is it a prison sentence. Genetics *can* play a role in illness. However, in the case of autoimmune and other chronic disorders, genes are merely a fraction of a single puzzle piece. There are so many reasons that people get sick that aren't gene-related on any level.

While any talk of genetics sounds impressive, don't be fooled. Do not let yourself go down this road of believing you are to blame for your illness. And if you've already gone miles down that dark path during your years of seeking answers, come back to the light! The reason that so many conditions appear to be inherited is that pathogens and pollutants are passed down from parent to child. On top of which, family members are often exposed to the same environmental factors simply because they live and travel together.

So if both you and your mother suffer from Hashimoto's, it's not because thyroiditis "runs in the family"—in the traditional understanding of the expression. A more realistic scenario is that your mother contracted EBV at some point in her life, before you were born. When you were conceived, she passed this strain of the thyroid virus on to you, and your father passed on ancient mercury inherited from his own parents. Then when you were a small child, you and your mother were both exposed to a pesticide application in your home, which took a toll on your immune systems. And because you and your mother were both under a lot of stress, perhaps due to strained family finances, lived with elevated levels of toxic heavy metals, and ate the same diet of unproductive foods such as ham omelets and canola-fried corn fritters, that virus had a chance to continue to flourish in your livers and eventually your thyroids. Your mother's thyroid problems and other EBV symptoms would have surfaced earlier, because she'd had the virus for longer. Your health issues would have developed later, as the virus moved at its own rate through your body, so it wouldn't have been evident that the two of you were experiencing triggers side by side. Genetics didn't enter into the equation at all.

Until medical communities accept the pathogenic and environmental factors involved, they won't be able to assist people in truly recovering from thyroid and other chronic illnesses.

This is important to remember in the coming years, as the genetic theory explodes. We haven't seen anything yet when it comes to blaming health problems on the very fiber of one's being. When you come back to this book in ten years, it will look like everything you're reading here is outdated, because genetics will have become the prevailing explanation for chronic health issues.

Convincing as it may sound, it won't be the real answer—what you're reading here will still be far more advanced. Gene blame is a joker's game where everybody walks away a loser. At the same time that you hear in the future that genes explain everything, if you look around, illness and suffering will be on the rise like never before. Not only will it keep research from pursuing the truth; gene blame itself will be a seed of destruction to immune systems for generations to come. That is, unless the truth in this book gets out. If experts start acknowledging the pathogens and pollutants that are really to blame, only then can true progress be made. (For more on the real factors behind illness, see "Great Mistake 7: Ignoring the Unforgiving Four.")

Funding is critical to which way this goes. Look at what funding has done for certain areas of life. Our children today can play the most mind-bogglingly advanced video games, for example, developed by companies flush with capital, while at the same time, these kids may suffer from mysterious asthma, acne, other skin conditions, sinus problems, insomnia, celiac disease, stomachaches, anxiety, depression, aches and pains, allergies, even thyroid problems, and a chronic stuffy nose—all issues where the answers are undiscovered, because that's not where the funding is.

Genetic funding is huge because the topic of genetics is an attractive lure, so that's where we see the headlines. One news item you might have read is that genes can be turned on and off depending on environmental exposures. This theory is not entirely inaccurate—it just doesn't happen to explain chronic illness. When environment plays a role in illness, it's not because the exposure has an effect on a gene, which creates someone's symptoms. It's because the environmental exposure breaks down someone's immune system and feeds viruses such as EBV. As I said, a person gets sick because of an overburdened immune system due to outside factors, whether they're passed down through the bloodline, encountered in the womb, or exposure happens after birth. Whether genes are turned on, off, or sideways, the Unforgiving Four factors you'll read about in the next chapter are the real explanation behind the epidemic of chronic illness. The gene world is going to become an unstoppable monster machine that will consume everybody's common sense.

And because outside factors are to blame for illness, this means you can protect yourself from them—which was the subject of my book *Medical Medium Life-Changing Foods: Save Yourself and the Ones You Love with the Hidden Healing Powers of Fruits and Vegetables*. The gene blame game, on the other hand, makes people feel like their own destruction comes from within themselves. When someone is suffering from a disease and told it's genetic, it can almost make that person feel like giving

up instantly and waiting to hear on the news someday that the cure has been found. This takes them down a darkened, hopeless path, longing for science to someday answer their prayers with a genetic miracle discovery that will never come because that's not where the real insights await.

Think of all the women getting tested to see if they're at genetic risk for breast cancer. The theory that the BRCA1 and BRCA2 genes are indicators that someone will develop breast cancer is causing women to have double mastectomies—an incredibly painful process—when the truth is that more women without BRCA gene mutations develop breast cancer than women with the gene mutations. Breast cancer is not caused by genes; as we looked at in Part I, it is almost always caused by EBV. Funding of EBV research, not genetics, is what will finally curb the breast cancer epidemic—and the thyroid illness epidemic.

It's so easy to be hoodwinked by the genetic theory of chronic illness, because there are some truly dazzling aspects of DNA and heredity. Don't let this extraordinary discovery be used against you, though. When it goes so far as to make you feel doomed to a certain health fate, dependent on a one-in-a-million chance of getting better, or at fault for feeling unwell, beware that gene blame is one of those runaway trains that will take you far from where you're meant to be.

CHAPTER 16

Great Mistake 7: Ignoring the Unforgiving Four

The four outside factors that are the real problems behind chronic and mystery illness—factors that I call the Unforgiving Four—are radiation, the viral explosion, DDT, and toxic heavy metals. Ignoring these is a Great Mistake that's not to be overlooked. (For more on any of these, see *Medical Medium Life-Changing Foods*.)

Radiation from the world's nuclear disasters such as Fukushima, Hiroshima, and Chernobyl has not gone away. That radiation still falls on us from the sky and will continue to long into the future. Plus, historical radiation mistakes such as overexposure and fluoroscopes continue to affect us with the radiation they passed along.

Even today, new radiation exposure is a concern. For one, more protective measures need to be taken during X-rays—we're still not conservative enough in this area. Also, that X-rays suddenly went digital should raise our eyebrows and make us ask what was discovered about the old X-rays' effects that made digital the safer option. In the future, even better, more streamlined techniques will be needed and developed.

It's not just X-rays where radiation is a problem. When flying, for example, there are more ways to be exposed to radiation than ever before. For one,

there's the Fukushima radiation in the atmosphere. And yet radiation as a health threat is swept under the carpet, practically ignored on all accounts.

As I mentioned earlier in the book, in a bit less than 5 percent of thyroid disease, radiation is the cause. That's because major radiation exposure overheats and practically cooks the gland itself—essentially giving the thyroid radiation burn.

And whether it gets to this point of injuring the gland or not, radiation also suppresses the immune system—both the thyroid's individual immune system and the body's overall immune system—which opens the door for EBV to take advantage of the thyroid, as well as for all sorts of other illnesses to take hold in the body.

The **viral explosion** is what explains so much of chronic illness today. While you've learned about EBV's destructiveness in this book, other viruses in the human herpesvirus (HHV) family such as shingles, cytomegalovirus (CMV), HHV-6, HHV-7, and the undiscovered HHV-10, HHV-11, and HHV-12 are also running through the population and taking people down.

The neurological symptoms of our time—brain fog, memory loss, tinnitus, frozen shoulder, migraines, deafening, tingles, numbness, neuropathy, neuralgia, muscle spasms, twitches, cramps, restless legs syndrome, anxiety, depression—not to mention health challenges such as Hashimoto's, Graves', ME/CFS, Lyme disease, fibromyalgia, RA, MS, lupus, Ehlers-Danlos syndrome, sarcoidosis, edema, and hepatitis C, to name just a few, will all be traced back to the viral explosion. As we looked at in Chapter 6, "Thyroid Cancer," 98 percent of cancers, too, will be traced back to a virus in combination with at least one type of toxin.

And as these viruses spread, they mutate, becoming even more pernicious. That is, it's not gene mutations causing the epidemic of health problems, as researchers suspect; it's hundreds of viral mutations.

These viruses don't get anywhere near the amount of attention they should, because they're difficult to detect and so misunderstood. Since Lyme disease is thought to be bacterial, for example, research directs itself away from viruses— which is the exact opposite of what would help. Ignoring the viral explosion comes at the cost of not finding the answers behind chronic illness.

DDT is similarly hidden from view—though in this case, it's because we're led to believe its dangers fall squarely in the past. The truth is that this once-popular pesticide, long since banned in many areas of the world, has not left us. Not only does it survive in the environment, which means it can make it into our food supply; it's also passed along from generation to generation. As enlightened as we've become about harmful chemicals, DDT's cousins are still in active use in the form of modern-day pesticides, herbicides, and fungicides that we encounter on conventional produce, use in our yards, and even spray in our homes, even though you'll find a skull and crossbones on some of those labels.

DDT is dangerous because it can break down the liver, feed viruses such as EBV, and weaken the immune system, opening the door so pathogens and other contaminants can take advantage. Though yet again, because it's passed down through family lines, it disguises itself as a genetic weakness, so DDT no longer gets any attention.

The theme of these Unforgiving Four is out of sight, out of mind. **Toxic heavy metals** are no exception. We can't see the copper, arsenic, cadmium, lead, nickel, mercury, aluminum, steels, and alloys that enter our systems through pesticides, herbicides, fungicides, DDT, pharmaceuticals such as antibiotics, and our bloodlines, so they must not be hurting us—or so the reasoning goes. If only this were true.

On their own, these toxic heavy metals wreak havoc when they're not detoxed. They are the ultimate food for pathogens, plus they drain the immune system. Over time, the metals oxidize and leach byproduct and residue, staining and damaging tissue in the body with this toxic runoff, which is more refined and processed than the metals in their raw state, making them easier for pathogens to consume. (Think of heavy metal runoff like a trough of pig slop.)

In combination, heavy metals are even worse—they form reactive alloys where the two or more metals bind to each other and set each other off at the same time. Like contraindicated medications, their reaction is bad news for your body, further weakening both the general immune system and the thyroid's individual immune system, allowing for viruses like EBV to build the army that causes illnesses such as thyroid disease to take hold.

As sobering as this information is, the Unforgiving Four don't spell doom—not nearly. With these factors, it's all about awareness, which is why ignoring them is a Great Mistake. When you know to look out for these in your daily life, and you know how to detox them using the techniques that I offer in the Medical Medium books, you don't have to live in fear.

CHAPTER 17

Great Mistake 8: It's All in Your Head

When you're ill with chronic symptoms, it can already feel crazy-making. Before discovering the Unforgiving Four, you may have asked yourself why you'd been sidelined as you watched friends and loved ones carry on life as usual. What was it that stuck you in bed on a sunny Saturday while your neighbor had to take your kid to soccer practice because you weren't well enough to drive? The hidden nature of chronic illnesses' causes can make it feel almost like you live inside an invisible fence.

This hiddenness and invisibility make your situation a mystery to others, too—from doctors to colleagues to the family members who rely on you. This makes it even worse. Because the answers aren't yet out there in the mainstream about what causes chronic health issues such as hypothyroidism and Hashimoto's, when lab tests and imaging and exams come back with no answers, it's much more rare for others to question the diagnostics than it is for them to question you.

Why are you still *sick?* they may ask you. *When will you get better?* And then, the more probing questions: *Are you sure this isn't just some childhood trauma resurfacing as a cry for attention? Have you tried focusing on something besides yourself, like a new hobby? Can't you just cheer up? Push yourself a little harder in life?* What they're getting at is this: *It's all in your head. Psychosomatic. Imaginary. Snap out of it.*

If only these people knew the depth of your suffering and the depth of your will to get better. The truth is that it probably scares them to see you ill. It makes them think it could happen to them, too, or that they'll lose you—so they make themselves feel better by saying you made it up. All we can really do is feel sorry for them, because telling you that you've made up your illness is one of the greatest mistakes of all time.

This idea got its real start in the late 1940s, when those droves of women we talked about earlier started to visit the doctor with fatigue, low energy, depression, brain fog, aches and pains, hair loss, unnatural weight gain, hot flashes, and anxiety. Because there was nothing in the medical textbooks to explain this epidemic, it was thought of as "crazy women syndrome." Women who were poor and reported feeling unwell were considered lazy; women who were wealthy and reported feeling unwell were considered bored. It was a new version of labeling women hysterical—and I don't mean funny. (By the way, all those historical cases of hysteria, which were blamed on the uterus, were actually mercury poisoning from the quicksilver remedies of the day.) After about a decade of "crazy women syndrome" as the prevailing wisdom, theories about hormonal imbalance and menopause entered the scene, and the hormone trend train took off.

I wish I could say that the "It's all in your head" reasoning stayed behind. As you know too well, it's still with us. Women and men, young and old, continue to get the message that they've somehow imagined their symptoms. Sometimes it's not even words that say it, only a look or a tone of voice. The doubt is unmistakable, though.

It drives people to visit the psychiatrist, looking for reasons why they'd be holding themselves back in life, wondering if they have a personality disorder that's making them act like they're sick. It's very common for these people to hear that their anxiety and depression are causing their symptoms. In reality, anxiety and depression themselves are common symptoms

(not causes) of chronic illness—because, as we looked at in Chapter 5, viral neurotoxins and heavy metals interfere with brain activity.

Even if you've now found a compassionate practitioner who believes your symptoms have a real, physical cause, that old hurt of once being told you'd made up your suffering may still be with you, and that's understandable. There is tremendous grief in what this message might have cost you—years on psychological pharmaceuticals, dignity in your relationships, or even relationships themselves. It's a Great Mistake that has ended marriages and caused children to turn on their parents (and vice versa) out of frustration and misunderstanding about why they couldn't get better. The "It's all in your head" stigma is the ultimate intuition destroyer, causing people to lose trust in their own judgment.

When this idea remains in circulation, it hurts everyone involved. It isolates the people who are suffering and prevents the people in their lives from pursuing the real answers. I hope to God that this becomes a mistake of the past soon.

CHAPTER 18

Great Mistake 9: You Created Your Illness

Talk about an intuition destroyer. If you've ever been made to feel like you created, attracted, or manifested your illness with your thoughts, karma, or energy, it's time to free yourself of this notion once and for all. You did not create your illness. You did not manifest your illness. You did not attract your illness. You do not deserve to be sick. Your fears and fixations did not bring your suffering to you. Your illness is not your fault. When you believe that you're to blame, you get cut off from the self-trust you need to navigate life—and to heal.

"You created your illness" is a new, hip, repackaged version of "It's all in your head." It's also more deceptive, because this theory does acknowledge that your physical symptoms are real. So it mixes truth and validation (you're suffering) with untruth and blame (you brought it upon yourself), leaving you to wonder where one ends and the other begins. Remember this: you did not bring it upon yourself!

Listen, nobody wants to be sick. That's just not how it works. Anybody who tells you otherwise is really saying, "I don't know what's wrong with you. I wish I did. I wish I could help you. The best I can do is to offer this theory."

Nobody has a fear of healing. If the reasoning were true that your fears become your reality, then there wouldn't be one healthy person—because everyone's afraid of getting sick. Nobody has a subconscious desire to be pinned to the couch with debilitating fatigue and muscle pain. Nobody secretly wishes to gain weight, lose hair, and deal with heart palpitations, feverishness, depression, anxiety, injuries that won't heal, insomnia, dizziness, and brain fog.

And yet the message that so many people, especially the younger generations, are getting now is that they create their own reality with their thoughts and feelings, so they're responsible for anything negative that comes their way. They hear that if their lives aren't perfect, it's because they're doing something wrong, and they're not spiritually connected enough. It's even to the point where they're told that a wrong they committed in a past life could explain why they're paying in the form of physical suffering in this one. How do I respond to this? That is simply not true.

Now, I don't want to discount the miraculous power of thoughts, intentions, and affirmations.

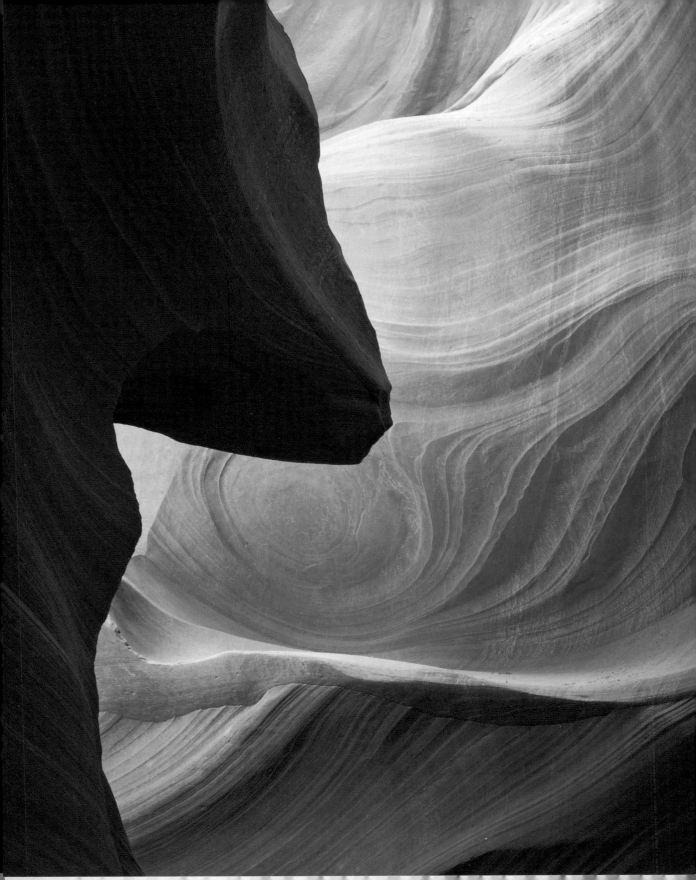

PART III

THYROID RESURRECTION

CHAPTER 19

Time to Rebuild Your Body

By now, you've gotten the point that to move on with your life, you want to get rid of the thyroid virus: Healing your thyroid and the rest of your body is all about saying good-bye to EBV. Getting your immune system back is all about getting past EBV. Leaving your symptoms behind is all about eradicating EBV.

Or is it? Here's the interesting part: As much as you want to lower your EBV levels and render it inactive, it shouldn't be your goal to get rid of every last EBV cell in your body. That's right—you only want to get rid of about 90 percent of the virus.

That remaining 10 percent of dormant EBV in your body serves as a constant reminder to your immune system to stay on alert. As we looked at in Chapter 3, "How the Thyroid Virus Works," there are over 60 varieties of the virus. Just because you've gotten past one bout of it doesn't mean you can't catch another—and this is not one of those times in life when you want to collect them all! I'm sure you'll agree that one go-round with EBV is more than enough. So with every new environment you enter, every new intimate relationship you begin—the times when you may encounter various strains of EBV—you want to make sure your body is fierce and ready to destroy any new Epstein-Barr viral cells. What gives you this edge

is holding on to a little of the conquered, dormant EBV variety you already have.

Think of your immune system like a fire department, ready, willing, and able to handle any issues that put your health in danger. Now imagine that fire department never gets any calls. A couple of years go by, and not one incident needs its attention. If this happens, the firefighters will grow complacent and lazy. They'll start *expecting* not to get any calls. They'll take days off, get lax with training, put all their energy into creating elaborate chili recipes and fried chicken dishes.

Now what happens if one night, after staying out late at a bar, drinking too much, and eating a pile of buffalo wings, the firefighters wake up to the alarm bell ringing? First, they'll scramble, struggling to run through the mental checklist that's supposed to be second nature. Still a little hungover and in shock that they're being summoned to an emergency, they'll slowly cobble together the gear and equipment that's meant to be laid out perfectly for maximum efficiency. Once they get to the fire truck, they'll find that the battery's dead from not being used. When they finally get it charged up, they'll rush to the fire, only to find that there was a leak in the water tank, and the hose is bone-dry. By now, the fire will be raging. If they'd been ready, they could have gotten to the fire early, put out the flames, and saved the house and the people who lived there with no problem.

That's your immune system—you want it in shape and at the ready. That fraction of defeated EBV keeps your immune system trained and on its toes instead of eating pizza in front of the TV every night.

FINDING YOUR FOOTING

You don't need to do anything special to make sure you keep a little dormant EBV. You still want your focus to be taming the virus, and that's what this portion of the book is all about. What's important is knowing what's going on behind the scenes so that you don't worry about still seeing those past-infection EBV antibodies show up on your blood tests. When you've been doing everything in this section of the book, the EBV in your system is dormant and defeated, beaten to a pulp by your antiviral measures. (Also don't worry if you don't see antibodies on blood tests; as we discussed, testing is not definitive.)

Don't lose faith if it takes a while to feel like yourself again. The healing timeline is different for everyone. If you haven't been ill for very long, you could be back in business in as little as three weeks. If you've been dealing with your symptoms for longer, you could be looking at three months, six months, or even a couple of years until you're truly back on your feet.

During that time, you'll feel better and better, leaving certain symptoms behind as others hang on for a little while longer, so that you're able to feel that sense of progress. Even if it's two steps forward and one step back at times, remember that this is a natural part of healing. When you're climbing a rock wall, you're not always going up, up, up. Sometimes you need to make a move sideways or a little down to find the right foothold

that will put you on the path to the top. Find a compassionate practitioner, and tell them about your mission.

Don't be discouraged if you've been sick for 30 years, and you know you have a lot of healing to do. From discovering the information in this book alone, you've set yourself on that upward path. Every now and then as you're moving along, take a moment to look back and remind yourself how far you've come.

When you're working on your health naturally and building up your immune system with the right foods and healthy practices, your thyroid will start to improve all on its own as the EBV ebbs. What's better, the rest of your body will improve, too. Your liver, your lymphatic system, your nerves, your circulation—with the right TLC, you can rebuild your body and reclaim your life

YOUR TIME TO HEAL

Given that testing isn't definitive, you may still be unsure if you're living with the thyroid virus. The good news is that it doesn't hurt to help protect your thyroid. Whether it turns out that Epstein-Barr is targeting your gland and causing your symptoms, or there's another reason you're suffering, the information to come can do wonders for your health. It always helps to detox heavy metals and other toxins, cleanse pathogens and their waste products, boost your immune system, and support your thyroid. After all the love and protection your body has given you over the years, it's time for it to feel the love right back.

Following a special chapter for those of you who've lost a thyroid to surgery or radioactive iodine treatments, let's look at how to clean up your symptoms, conquer your illnesses, tame EBV, and revive your thyroid—and with this reclaim your healthy self.

CHAPTER 20

Life without a Thyroid

What if you don't have a thyroid anymore? People without their thyroids often feel like they don't get to have a thyroid book privilege—like they don't get to learn about thyroid healing, because it doesn't apply to them. I'm here to say otherwise.

Over the decades, I've known so many people who thought of their thyroids as past-tense stories. They came to me for other health reasons, and yet I would ask, "Why don't we talk a bit about your thyroid?"

Almost always, these people would be shocked. What was there to say? The gland was gone, nothing could be done anymore, and that was that, they thought. The health professionals and experts they'd consulted had never been able to explain what had happened in the first place to create problems with the thyroid; they had been left without answers about what had caused them to lose a piece of themselves. These people didn't believe they were even allowed to consider talking about their thyroids again in a way that could have anything to do with improving their health.

As we talked more, they discovered what had really happened inside their bodies to result in the thyroid nodule, cyst, cancer, or hyper-thyroidism that eventually led doctors to want to remove or "kill off" the gland. They realized that even without their thyroids, the thyroid virus could still be active and causing symptoms, since EBV resides in other parts of the body, too. Not only that, they learned that their thyroids still held meaning. The thyroid remained a piece of them that had potential.

If you've had all or part of your thyroid surgically removed, or if you've undergone a radioactive iodine treatment to destroy the gland, don't feel left out, as though you don't get to have your own journey to health.

First of all, there's that important detail to remember: The symptoms labeled as "hypothyroid symptoms" are almost always viral, not related to a deficiency of thyroid hormones. So when you get EBV to retreat, the symptoms go away, too—even if you don't have a thyroid.

There's a second critical piece of information you need: your body still believes you have your entire thyroid.

It's like this: If your house is robbed, it stays standing. The walls are still there, and you still have your home. Same with your thyroid. When part of your thyroid is removed, there's still tissue remaining around the edges; those "walls" are still there. Your body still considers you as having a thyroid.

And when your house is knocked down—when thyroid surgery is more invasive, or when radioactive iodine kills the tissue—you still have the home's foundation. You can build on what you have.

Even if that foundation is dug out, the spirit of the home remains. You still have the address; you can still send and receive mail—just like the body can still function as though the thyroid is in place, even if all or part of it is gone.

You must consciously connect to this truth, because it's your body's way of helping you survive, adapt, and heal. It means that the rest of your endocrine system works as it's meant to, in a state of homeostasis, and continues to support the thyroid.

Why would you want your body to continue to support the thyroid gland when it's not there anymore? Because even if you heard that your surgery removed the gland entirely or your radioactive iodine treatment killed it off completely, the overwhelming probability is that you still have functional thyroid tissue left. Many people who've been told their thyroid is completely gone actually have 30 to 40 percent of their thyroid tissue remaining. And even if you have as little as one percent of your thyroid tissue, it can still produce a small amount of the thyroid hormones T4 and T3, which are beneficial to your healing, as well as the undiscovered thyroid hormones R5 and R6 that are involved with sending out the thyroid's radio-like frequencies that promote homeostasis throughout the body. On top of which, as we looked at in Chapter 4, your adrenals will also produce their own tailor-made steroid blend to help replace any diminished thyroid hormones.

No matter how much or how little thyroid tissue you have, it is working for you. It may even be working better for you than someone who has an entire thyroid that's only able to do 40 percent of its work due to a long-term thyroid virus infection that has caused a lot of scarring over time. When you're missing thyroid tissue, the living thyroid tissue you have left amps up its game. The cells learn to adapt, become stronger, and take on more responsibility, shielding themselves from future attacks of EBV because their numbers are limited. They do this by communicating with the thyroid's personalized immune system, sending out distinctive radio-like frequencies to these special lymphocytes to indicate that they need extra protection.

If you've been treated with radioactive iodine, you can work to chelate this substance with healing foods. Small and even tiny amounts of Atlantic dulse and spirulina in your regular diet especially help to remove radioactive iodine from the thyroid over time, bringing what's left of the gland back to life in a balanced manner they don't over-revive the gland to the point of hyperactivity. The beneficial, bioactive iodine in dulse and spirulina can bind on to the leftover radioactive isotopes, driving them out of the thyroid, at the same time driving out old, unwanted radiation that's made it into the thyroid or other parts of the body from everyday exposure. This trace iodine content is also beneficial to the thyroid overall. (For more on iodine, see the next chapter.) It's best to supplement these foods with other anti-radiation foods, too, some of which are included in Chapter 22, "Powerful Foods, Herbs, and Supplements for Healing," and many more of which you can find in my book *Medical Medium Life-Changing Foods*.

With the proper care, your thyroid tissue can regenerate just enough so that your thyroid function improves over time. So as you read this portion of the book, know that it all applies to you, too. Get in the mind-set that you have a thyroid that's there and working hard for you, one that you want to protect and nurture, and you'll be on your way to healing.

CHAPTER 21

Common Misconceptions and What to Avoid

As you saw in Part II, "The Great Mistakes in Your Way," so much of safeguarding your health is knowing what *not* to listen to. In the quest to prevent and get people better from chronic illness, health authorities have put so many theories out there about what will offer relief. Sadly, the bulk of these ideas are at best a distraction, and at worst liable to make you sicker.

If you followed every piece of thyroid health advice out there, you'd be living life in a labyrinth—first turning this way, then that way, coming upon dead end after dead end, never able to see where you're going with any perspective. Not only is it exhausting and disheartening; it wastes the precious time you could be using to heal.

Consider this chapter the orange cones and caution tape blocking off those dead ends. When you know what to avoid, you can find your way out of the maze.

CONCERNS ABOUT IODINE

Many people are concerned about iodine in relation to hypothyroidism and Hashimoto's thyroiditis. To understand whether iodine is beneficial or detrimental for someone with an underactive and/or inflamed thyroid, we have to think about it in the context of what the undiscovered cause of the thyroid problem is in the first place: the Epstein-Barr virus.

Iodine is a disinfectant, effective at killing both viruses and bacteria. You've probably used it or heard of it being used as an antiseptic to clean wounds and prevent infection. When high-quality iodine is in someone's system, either through diet or supplementation, it applies this same germ-fighting ability. This also means that someone with an iodine *deficiency* is more vulnerable to bacterial and viral infections. So if you have a thyroid infection of EBV that's causing hypothyroidism and/or Hashimoto's, you don't want to be iodine deficient, because it can translate to greater EBV susceptibility, which equates to thyroid illness susceptibility.

Why is there so much confusion about iodine and the thyroid? Because when iodine reaches the thyroid, it kills off virus cells at an accelerated rate, which can in turn temporarily elevate inflammation. Those patients for whom EBV is only causing a mild hypothyroid can often

available from everyday food sources, so we're all high in it, able to recoup it quickly, and not at risk for becoming deficient. It's also very common to be high in that toxic copper, so if the lesser zinc supplement is cleansing you of it, it's doing you a favor. Of course, it's still best to go with high-quality, preservative-free, liquid zinc sulfate.

Another zinc trend has been gaining popularity lately. This one claims that if you can taste the zinc in a zinc supplement, it means you don't need zinc anymore. That's not correct. If you've been taking zinc for a few weeks or months and suddenly you begin to taste it, this does not mean you suddenly don't need it. Or if you're suffering from a sore throat and try a bit of zinc to see if that will help you, and you determine that you don't need it because the zinc taste is strong, you'll deprive yourself of an opportunity to end the symptom early. Delivering some liquid zinc sulfate supplement to a throat made raw by bacterial or viral infection can be the difference between suffering and seeing the light of healing.

Many factors affect how zinc tastes at a given moment, including prescription medications and dozens of foods, drinks, and their combinations. Drinking herbal tea with lemon and honey, for example, will intensify the taste of zinc taken afterward for at least four to six hours. Drinking coffee will do the opposite, its bitterness overwhelming the taste buds and making them less sensitive to detecting zinc. So whether or not you can taste zinc is an inaccurate gauge of whether or not you're deficient. A better determination is if you have a thyroid problem or any other chronic symptom or illness that sends you to the doctor for help. Zinc deficiency is rampant. As with iodine, zinc deficiency can even be passed along at birth.

It's tough to get enough zinc from food alone anymore. Even the best organic farms tend to be missing this mineral from their soil, in part due to the elevated levels of toxic heavy metals that fall from the sky, altering the pH balance of the soil, depleting soil-borne microorganisms, and reacting negatively with the soil's trace minerals such as zinc. This means that while pumpkin seeds, which are celebrated for their zinc content, can be supportive, along with certain foods noted for zinc in Chapter 22, if you're dealing with a symptom or condition, then supplementing with high-quality, liquid zinc sulfate will offer you an important immune boost. Consult with your practitioner about the right dosage for you. And remember: zinc fear will only get in the way of your healing.

"GOITROGENIC" FEAR

Cruciferous vegetables such as kale, cauliflower, broccoli, cabbage, collard greens, and more have gotten a bad name lately. So have other completely innocent foods such as peaches, pears, strawberries, and spinach. Don't believe the hype that these foods that contain so-called goitrogens are harmful to the thyroid.

The concept of goitrogens—that is, goiter-causing compounds—has been blown way out of proportion. In the first place, none of these foods contains enough goitrogens to be a health concern. Secondly, the goitrogens present in these foods are bonded to phytochemicals and amino acids that stop the goitrogens from doing harm. Even if you ate 100 pounds of broccoli in a day (which is impossible), the goitrogens still wouldn't be a problem for your health.

Your thyroid actually relies on these foods. They contain some of the nutrients that the gland needs the most, which is why cruciferous vegetables get special treatment in the next chapter. So don't pay this goitrogenic food fad any mind! Otherwise, you'll be missing out on a major opportunity for health.

WHAT NOT TO EAT

No matter what food belief system you subscribe to, whether high-protein, vegetarian, or the like, it's a good idea to remove eggs, dairy products, gluten, canola oil, soy, corn, and pork from your diet while you're dealing with a thyroid issue. It's not that these foods *cause* inflammation, which is the theory you might have heard. Rather, these foods feed EBV—the thyroid virus—and then the EBV creates inflammation. With these foods in your diet, the virus can continue to grow and prosper, which means that your thyroid and viral symptoms can continue to stick around. (You'll find even more information on what makes these foods problematic for someone with chronic symptoms or illness in the first two books of this Medical Medium series.)

One Egg Away

You know how delicious a fried egg is? EBV thinks so, too. Eggs are the top food to avoid with EBV, because they're the virus's number one food source. If you broke an egg into a petri dish and then introduced active EBV cells, the virus would proliferate rapidly. It doesn't matter if they're organic, free-range eggs—they're still problematic if you have EBV. And don't be confused by labels that claim the eggs are hormone-free. That only means they don't contain additional hormones; they're still filled with natural hormones that EBV loves.

If someone is in Stage One of the virus, all it could take is one more omelet or scrambled egg to launch the EBV into Stage Two's full-blown mononucleosis. This is true at any stage of the virus—at any given time, someone may only be one egg away from EBV's next phase of attack.

Listen, I know how tempting eggs are, and how many sources will tell you they're a perfect food. Again, this is not about any sort of food belief system. I'm not anti-egg; they do have nutrition that works well for some people. It's just that when you're dealing with any sort of thyroid condition or other viral issue, the problematic aspects of eggs outweigh the benefits, and they will work against all the other steps you take to try to heal. When you're swayed to indulge, remind yourself that eggs are part of the reason EBV has become so strong and widespread in the population. While you're working to get your health back, stay away from them.

Pass on the Cheese, Please

Dairy protein is EBV's second-favorite part of your diet. If you're dealing with the symptoms or conditions we've looked at in this book, it's best to avoid all dairy while you're trying to get better. This includes cheese, milk, butter, yogurt, cream, kefir, ghee—you get the idea. I wish I could say the opposite, because I know how fun dairy is. I wish I could tell you cheese pizza with a fried egg on top is the best thing you could eat for your thyroid. What I hope for more is your healing. My job is to have your back, so I have to tell you the truth, which is that even the best-sourced dairy from the happiest pasture-raised, grass-fed cows is going to hold you back if you're trying to get better from EBV and thyroid illness.

Gluten Mystery Misery

Luckily, people are catching on that gluten is a problematic food for those with chronic health issues. So many more gluten-free products and recipes are available today than just a few years ago, and it's no longer so isolating to say that you're passing on wheat. The reason gluten is coming off of menus and ingredient lists is not because what's wrong with it is widely understood, though. Rather, it's been process of elimination that's shown many doctors and patients that life without wheat in the diet can significantly improve someone's health.

The reason to avoid wheat gluten when you have one of the chronic issues in this book is not because gluten contains mycotoxins or is simply an inflammatory food, like the theories out there say. Rather, as with the other foods in this list, it's because gluten fuels pathogens, including EBV. (When it's gluten from GMO wheat, it's even worse.) When you have an EBV infection and you eat a piece of bread, the EBV has a feeding frenzy, giving off its waste product of neurotoxins in the process and setting off symptoms such as tingles and numbness, headaches, migraines, fatigue, brain fog, blurry eyes, aches and pains, and mood swings. Taking gluten out is one step toward starving EBV, which is why you'll see so many health improvements when you avoid it.

No Canola in Your Granola

This is another instigator, and the particular trouble here is that it's often represented as a health food. You've probably heard the claims that canola is good for you. Know that if you have EBV, canola is going to work against you. Not only should you eliminate it from your own kitchen, you should take care when eating out to make sure that your food is not prepared with either canola or a canola oil blend. Also check the labels of packaged foods, and leave those that contain canola on the shelf. Otherwise, you'll risk damage to your immune system, organs, and linings—all while this substance fuels EBV.

Corn Games

In the early days, corn was our friend. It was a healthy, amazing source of nourishment for us. Then, in the late 1930s and the 1940s, use of pesticides, herbicides, and fungicides on corn crops grew at an alarming rate. As you've read in this book, these sorts of chemical solutions are fuel for EBV, so when people ate this corn that was laden with toxic substances such as DDT, it started to feed EBV. As corn continued to get treated with enormous amounts of these chemicals, EBV started to identify corn itself with these toxins, because they were together all the time.

This continued through the decades, with conventionally grown corn feeding EBV . . . and then GMO corn arrived. That's when the corn games really got started, with genetic modification altering corn in a way that suited viruses. At this point, unfortunately, even organic corn grown from non-GMO seed is likely contaminated and can still trigger health conditions.

You don't need to fear corn. Just be cautious and consider where you are with your symptoms and conditions when corn and dishes made with corn oil, cornmeal, and the like are offered to you. As much as you can, avoid corn in its various forms, always saying "no" to conventional corn and skipping sneaky ingredients such as citric acid, high-fructose corn syrup, and grain alcohol (a common preservative in herbal tinctures). When you're not dealing with illness, it's okay to enjoy an organic corn on the cob, though keep it sparing. If you'd like, you can eat it alongside some of the healing foods from Chapter 22 to counter any ill effects.

Soy It Isn't So

Soy was also a relatively healthy food in years past—not as healthy as corn once was, though it still had plenty of benefits. Once again, overuse of pesticides and herbicides, along with GMO tampering, made soy crops unstable. The soybean of today is not the soybean of yesterday. It is altered now, a pathogen-feeding byproduct of what it used to be. While soy does not fuel viruses and bacteria on the same scale that corn does, it has the potential to get there.

One of the main problems with soy is its relatively high fat content, which harbors GMO information and high concentrations of pesticides and herbicides. Organic, non-GMO soy is what you want to look for, though there are no guarantees that it will be pure. If you love soy, try not to let it dominate your diet, and enjoy it sparingly instead. Whenever possible, opt for sprouted soy, which is lower in fat and therefore lower in concentrations of toxic chemicals.

Pork's Not Perfect

One of the issues with pork products is that they tend to have higher fat content than any other animal products, even if the pork is "lean" or "white meat." The other problem is the type of fat that pork contains. Though it may seem like typical animal fat, it in fact takes hours longer to disperse in the bloodstream after a meal—typically 12 to 16 hours, compared with the 3 to 6 hours other animal fats take to disperse.

Due to that long time it takes for pork fat to leave the bloodstream, if you eat sausage pizza for dinner and then have bacon the next morning, the prior evening's pork fat hasn't had a chance to exit your bloodstream before breakfast gives you a new dose. It means your blood doesn't get a chance to oxygenate between meals. With other sources of fat, such as other animal proteins, the time between dinner and breakfast is enough to at least give your body a break.

Oxygenation is key. When you're dealing with thyroid illness or another health condition, you don't want your bloodstream to have high fat content, particularly not for long periods of time. The higher the fat level in your bloodstream, the less oxygenated blood will be—and oxygen assists you with killing off bacteria and viruses such as EBV. Higher fat and less oxygen mean more of a chance for EBV and its pathogen cousins to thrive at your expense. Lower fat and more oxygen mean a better ability for your body to fight off EBV.

Pork fat also puts a burden on your liver, making it almost impossible for any heavy metals, pesticides, EBV cells, or viral waste matter that are present in your system to leave. Instead, these toxins get reabsorbed back into your organs, which can in turn hinder bodily functions such as the liver's conversion of thyroid hormones.

If you want to give your body the best chance to recuperate, keep your distance from bacon, sausage, ham, pork rinds, pork roasts, pork ribs, pork chops, pork tenderloins, pulled pork, processed pork products, and lard—tasty as they may be—while you're healing.

ONE DAY AT A TIME

I know it may feel overwhelming to leave behind the comforts of certain foods while you work on your healing. Keep in mind that you don't have to go cold turkey on ham and cheese sandwiches (or any of the other foods here). Back off the problematic foods little by little. Put a list of what you're trying to avoid on the fridge, as a reminder to yourself and those who live with you. Start with a new recipe or two from Chapter 24 to see what life is like without these foods.

One of the best ways to move forward is to fill your life with so many of the healing foods we'll look at in the next chapter that you simply don't have room in your fridge or on your plate for those that used to be a more regular part of your diet. I've seen people get so much joy out of focusing on these foods that any sense of loss about leaving behind old favorites vanishes. If you do feel that loss and those cravings—and rightfully so—you may find comfort in the chapter "Food for the Soul" in my book *Medical Medium Life-Changing Foods*.

Above all, know that I am right there with you as you make these transitions in your life. I believe in you 100 percent. I am there with you 100 percent. You can do this—you're not alone.

CHAPTER 22

Powerful Foods, Herbs, and Supplements for Healing

Your organs and glands need nourishment. On some level we know this—after all, we hear the term *brain food* all the time, and for good reason. In order to deal with our mile-a-minute lives, our brains need all kinds of fuel.

The thyroid needs to be fed, too. Especially when it's been depleted after weeks, months, or years of fighting the thyroid virus, your thyroid—this second brain of your body—is ready for nutrient therapy so it can restore itself. Plus, your nerves, immune system, liver, lymphatic system, adrenal glands, and, yes, brain, all need their share of support after going up against the thyroid virus, EBV. That's where this chapter comes in. It's all about giving your body the tools it needs to kill off the virus, repair the viral damage that's been done, and regenerate so you can have the best tomorrow.

Do I have to change my life overnight? you may ask yourself. Absolutely not. Consider this chapter a catalogue of all the options available to you, rather than a rule book. Incorporating these healing items into your life is all about creating a routine that's sustainable for *you*. What's most important is that you move forward in a way that works for you, so that you don't give up after three days—or before you even start—and decide you're not up to the task. You are absolutely up for this. Hang in there. Keep a light heart with it all. This isn't about adopting yet another food belief system; it's about finding what's best for you as an individual.

One of the challenges of healing from EBV is that as it begins to die off in certain parts of the body, the virus fights back by trying to start up second and even third rounds of infection. That's why, after a period of feeling better, you may develop new symptoms or a fresh wave of fatigue. Take heart that this is a natural part of healing, and that the more of these healing items you have in your life, the better positioned you'll be to shorten or prevent these extra viral cycles.

It's so important not to think of adding these items to your diet as a chore. Foods, herbs, and supplements are going to be your new best friends. These aren't the friends who drain and grate you, the ones whose calls you need to avoid for your sanity. These foods, herbs, and supplements are the friends who watch your back and are always there for you, no matter what. As you work to free yourself of EBV and bring your thyroid and the rest of your body back to health, these antiviral, antibacterial, tissue-repairing, immune-boosting, hormone-stabilizing, mood-enhancing, cleansing, transformative health restoratives will be the most loyal, committed supporters you could ask for. They truly are life-changing.

HEALING FOODS

Since you're your own health expert now, you're the one in the best position to evaluate which of the foods to come speak to your condition and symptoms. If you want to add all of them, go for it! If you want to take a more measured, realistic approach, think about picking three foods to concentrate on in your first week. Clip the list to your fridge as a reminder to bring a sizeable serving of each into your diet every day. The next week, pick three more foods, add them to your list, and incorporate them into your daily meals, too. This is not about eating a leaf of lettuce here or a slice of apple there. In order to see changes, you'll want to make sure you bring these healing foods into your life in quantity.

You can see how quickly those unproductive foods we looked at in the previous chapter can get edged out of your diet when you're filling up on these healing foods. In the next chapter, we'll look at a structure for how you may want to bring them into your life for maximum benefit. The chapter after that, "Thyroid Healing Recipes," offers delicious ways to prepare them. If you'd like to learn even more about the specific properties and benefits of these foods, you'll find lengthier features on them, along with more recipes, in my book *Medical Medium Life-Changing Foods*. And if the thought of eating fruit for health goes against what you've heard, check out the chapter "Fruit Fear" in *Medical Medium* to put those worries aside. Know this: cutting yourself off from fruit will cut you off from healing.

Arming Your Thyroid with Artichokes

Artichokes are some of your best allies when healing from the thyroid virus. Their hearts contain nutrients to support and restore your thyroid gland itself—notably, phytochemicals that communicate with the thyroid's frequency delivery system. These phytochemical compounds are undiscovered subgroups of isothiocyanates that work specifically with enzymes and amino acids in our bodies to enter into and support our immune systems and thyroids. These compounds support the production of the thyroid hormones we looked at earlier that remain undiscovered by medical research and science. These isothiocyanate subgroups also help to shrink nodules, tumors, and cysts by triggering an antitumor hormone that lies inside of human cells, even inside many nodules, tumors, and cysts, exposing the EBV that created them to our immune system. Further, these subgroups supplement the thyroid with tyrosine, a chemical needed to produce thyroid hormones. Plus, they help detox the liver of neurotoxins, dermatoxins, and the Unforgiving Four factors.

Artichoke leaves—that is, the "meat" you nibble off at the base of the artichoke scales—are armor for your thyroid. That's because the edible portion of artichoke leaves (technically, bracts) contains alkaloid compounds that send messages to specific parts of your immune system to guard your thyroid from invaders such as EBV. When EBV is already present in the thyroid, artichokes' nutrition acts as an anti-proliferative, helping to slow the virus's growth there. Bringing artichokes into your life is like giving your tender and precious thyroid its very own shield.

For guidance on how to prepare artichokes and incorporate them into your meals, see the recipes in Chapter 24. Beware that canned, bottled, and even some frozen artichoke hearts often contain citric acid, a corn-derived irritant, so you should soak them overnight to get rid of the preservative before eating.

Your Other Food Allies

When you combine artichokes with the foods in this list, you offer your body an amazing tool kit for recovery.

- **Aloe vera:** The gel from a fresh aloe leaf is a wonderful antiviral that also flushes toxins out of the bloodstream and body, helping to purge the liver specifically of toxins such as pesticides. Aloe supports the adrenals and draws radiation out of the thyroid.

- **Apples:** Anti-inflammatory for the thyroid because they starve EBV. When their pectin enters the digestive system, it releases phytochemicals that bind onto EBV, shrouding the virus cells so that they can't feed and proliferate.

- **Arugula:** Reduces nodules, tumors, and cysts in the thyroid (both cancerous and benign) and helps prevent EBV-related thyroid cancer in the first place. Arugula's phytochemical compounds enter into the thyroid, rejuvenating tissue there while reducing thyroid scar tissue. These compounds also push out old storage bins of thyroid medication from the liver.

- **Asparagus:** Cleanses the liver and spleen, strengthens the pancreas, and acts as an incredible supporter of the thyroid. Asparagus doesn't just inhibit the growth of EBV, it prohibits it. Phytochemicals in the skin and tips of the asparagus push back the virus and help stop it from reproducing. Asparagus also contains a pain-relieving alkaloid that acts as a gentle aspirin throughout the body. Try it raw in juice or steamed.

- **Atlantic sea vegetables (especially dulse and kelp):** Just as we put iodine on wounds, the iodine content of Atlantic sea vegetables such as dulse is an antiseptic for the thyroid—when it soaks into the gland, it becomes one of the thyroid's most powerful fighting mechanisms next to zinc. Luckily, dulse and other sea vegetables also contain some zinc. These two precious minerals at work together can stop a viral infection in the thyroid, bringing down thyroiditis (inflammation of the thyroid) in the process. Sea vegetables also help protect the thyroid from radiation's effects, remove radiation from the thyroid, and prevent thyroid cancer.

- **Avocados:** Contain phytochemicals that protect the lining of the digestive tract from EBV's cofactor, strep bacteria. Also contain an easily assimilable form of copper that helps balance T4 and T3 thyroid hormone production. Avocados' form of natural glucose calms sensitive nerves throughout the body that have been irritated by viral neurotoxins.

- **Bananas:** Provide amino acids and the right kind of potassium to rebuild neurotransmitters after they've been burnt out by EBV's neurotoxins. Also powerful for their antiviral, anti-inflammatory properties. A wonderful calcium source because the trees grow in calcium-rich soil, they're also a great tool for hypoglycemia, as they help balance blood sugar. Don't worry about the fad that says bananas have too much sugar. Their fruit sugar is actually critical brain food, plus it's bonded to the amino acids and minerals that give bananas their life-changing nutrition.

- **Basil:** This herb's antiviral abilities come in part from phytochemical compounds that can enter into the thyroid and slow down EBV cells' drilling action. Basil helps reduce nodules, cysts, and tumors, and holds anticancer compounds to help prevent thyroid cancer.

- **Berries:** Have a profound effect on the thyroid, notably because they are high in antioxidants that can act as a slow-down mechanism for accelerated thyroid tissue damage. Specific berries offer specific healing properties, as well. For example, blackberries help reduce the growth of nodules while they fortify and strengthen thyroid tissue. Raspberries are a great full-body detoxifying food, rich in antioxidants that specifically remove EBV's byproduct and other viral debris from the bloodstream, allowing for easier overall cleansing. Raspberries also tend to bind onto and remove impurities delivered to the intestinal tract by a liver burdened by viral waste

matter. (Wild blueberries have their own entry in this list.)

- **Cauliflower:** Often avoided by thyroid patients because it's labeled "goitrogenic," cauliflower is in fact one of your thyroid's best friends, as it helps the thyroid fight off EBV and contains trace mineral boron to support the entire endocrine system. Cauliflower also contains phytochemicals that can stop the thyroid from shrinking during the atrophy that can occur from long-term overmedication with prescription thyroid hormones.

- **Celery:** Strengthens hydrochloric acid in the gut and helps the liver produce bile to break down food. Provides mineral salts that are anti-EBV and help support the central nervous system with powerful electrolytes while they stabilize and support the adrenal glands. Celery has the ability to cleanse the thyroid of EBV toxins. Also bolsters the production of the thyroid hormone T3.

- **Cilantro**: A miracle worker for EBV. Critical for binding onto the toxic heavy metals such as mercury and lead that feed the virus. Also binds onto the EBV neurotoxins that, when loose in your system, can cause tingles and numbness, aches and pains, inflammation, depression, and anxiety.

- **Coconut:** Antiviral and anti-inflammatory, coconut kills EBV cells and reduces nodule growth.

Helps support the central nervous system from exposure to EBV neurotoxins. Try it as coconut oil, coconut butter, dried coconut (if it's unsweetened and unsulfured), coconut milk, and coconut water.

- **Cruciferous vegetables:** The rich sulfur content of these foods is a disinfectant and deterrent to EBV in the thyroid. Sulfur has a ghostlike quality, saturating the gland and creating a smoke-screen effect so the virus can't function well. At the same time, that sulfur helps revitalize the gland itself—contrary to the popular belief that these vegetables in the *Brassica* family are problematic for the thyroid. In order of importance, here are some of the best crucifers to bring into your life (find more on the first five individually in this list): cauliflower, kale, radishes, arugula, watercress, brussels sprouts, cabbage, broccoli, kohlrabi, collard greens, broccoli rabe, and mustard greens.

- **Cucumbers:** Strengthen the adrenals and kidneys and flush EBV neurotoxins out of the bloodstream. Hydrate the lymphatic system, especially the part based around the neck area (where the thyroid has its own immune system with specially assigned lymphocytes that seek out EBV cells), allowing for better cleansing of the thyroid. Cucumber hydration can slow down and even stop a fresh mononucleosis infection.

- **Dates:** Contain potassium, magnesium, and glucose that support your endocrine system. Dates help to purge the liver of debris often caused by EBV waste matter. They also trigger peristaltic action, helping the intestinal tract to squeeze and push out multiple varieties of waste that can burden the body when trying to heal.

- **Fennel:** High in vitamin C and other strong antiviral compounds to fight off EBV. Fennel seeds contain an aspirin-like compound with a deflating quality that acts as an anti-inflammatory to a thyroid flared up by EBV. This calming of the thyroid helps improve its hormone production.

- **Figs:** Grab on to toxins in the intestinal tract and drive them out of the body so you can heal. Also purge the liver of pesticides, old pharmaceuticals such as thyroid medications, and other waste, making the liver a less happy place for EBV to dwell.

- **Garlic:** Antiviral and antibacterial that defends against EBV by killing off virus cells. Also kills off strep, the EBV cofactor, allowing for fewer UTIs, sinus infections, and opportunities for SIBO. Helps flush toxic viral and bacterial waste out of the lymphatic system.

- **Ginger:** Helps with nutrient assimilation and relieves spasms associated with EBV and an overabundance of stress. Loaded with its own signature variety of bioavailable vitamin C, ginger is also a powerful antiviral against EBV. One of ginger's special qualities is its ability to bring the body out of a reactive state—which can happen easily when EBV is on the scene—by soothing nerves and muscles. Ginger helps bring balance and homeostasis to the thyroid, lifting it up if it's hypo and calming it down if it's hyper.

- **Hemp seeds:** Provide micronutrients and vital amino acids for your thyroid. Great for protecting the heart from EBV's biofilm byproduct that can gum up valves in the organ and create heart palpitations. Also great for fortifying the cardiovascular system. Help protect other parts of the body that get affected by EBV, including the eyes—for example, they help reduce eye floaters.

- **Kale:** High in specific alkaloids that protect against viruses such as EBV. Its phytochemicals can enter the thyroid, killing off pockets of EBV that start to develop there during the virus's early stages of occupying the gland.

- **Lemons and limes:** Improve digestion by raising levels of hydrochloric acid (good acid) in the gut. Tone the intestinal lining, cleanse the liver, and offer replenishing calcium to prevent osteoporosis when EBV prompts nodule formation throughout the body, which uses up calcium

stores. Lemons and limes also balance sodium levels in the blood, which allows for electrolytes to become active and improves the neurotransmitter activity that has been hampered by EBV neurotoxins causing brain fog and other neurological symptoms.

- **Lettuce** (especially butter leaf and romaine): Stimulates peristaltic action in the intestinal tract and helps cleanse EBV from the liver and lymphatic system. Blood cleansing and blood building. Holds trace mineral salts that support the adrenal glands, which ultimately supports the thyroid.

- **Mangoes**: Contain a tremendous amount of carotene to restore the spleen and liver, feed the brain, and purge the lymphatic system of EBV waste-matter toxins. Also provides bioactive magnesium and glucose that calm nerves to aid in sleep issues caused by EBV.

- **Maple syrup:** Holds dozens of trace minerals that fortify the brain and the rest of the nervous system, protecting them from oxidation due to heavy metal damage and EBV neurotoxins. Helps to build glycogen storage banks in the liver and brain to help balance blood sugar, which keeps the adrenals strong and stable so they can support the thyroid.

- **Nuts (especially walnuts, Brazil nuts, almonds, and cashews):** Hold trace minerals such as zinc, selenium, and manganese that are helpful in supporting the thyroid. Walnuts, for example, hold antiviral and antibacterial phytochemical compounds that inhibit EBV from proliferating in the liver, spleen, and thyroid.

- **Onions and scallions:** Another fantastic resource for their sulfur content's ability to confuse and knock down EBV while it nourishes the gland itself. As with cruciferous vegetables, that pungent quality is exactly what gives them their value. Onions are a big deal for fighting EBV—bottom line, a potent antiviral.

- **Oranges and tangerines:** Like lemons and limes, a rich source of calcium, which is vital when your body needs the mineral to block EBV from causing thyroid damage. Getting plenty of bioavailable calcium—the best source is citrus—prevents your body from needing to tap into the calcium reserves in your bones. Oranges' and tangerines' vitamin C content, too, is a tool against EBV, helping to revive the liver from EBV damage and purge the organ of fat and EBV debris, in the process helping you lose weight.

- **Papayas:** Restore the central nervous system from neurotoxin damage. Strengthen and rebuild hydrochloric acid in the gut. Their vitamin C content is an anti-EBV secret weapon and also helps cleanse and rebuild the liver. The phytochemical compounds in papayas that illuminate their rich, glowing, red-orange flesh have the ability to drive more sunlight into the thyroid itself when someone is outside enjoying a nice day. This additional sunlight absorption retards EBV's growth and its ability to twist and drill itself into a thyroid. Papayas also help stop thyroid atrophy.

- **Parsley:** Removes high levels of copper and aluminum, which feed EBV and in turn cause skin problems. Bolsters production of the thyroid hormone T3 by helping to feed and restore the thyroid.

- **Pears:** Revitalize and feed the liver while cleansing and purging the organ of pesticides and EBV waste matter. This process helps correct a sluggish liver so weight loss can occur. Very helpful in reducing insulin resistance, balancing blood sugar, and supporting the adrenals.

- **Pomegranates:** Help detox and cleanse the blood as well as the lymphatic system. Inhibit EBV and other viruses; break down nodules, tumors, and cysts throughout the body, including the thyroid; revitalize and rejuvenate thyroid tissue. Aid the adrenals. Help protect and clean the parathyroid gland.

- **Potatoes:** Frequently labeled as a "white" food that's devoid of nutrition, potatoes are actually one of the most powerful anti-EBV foods. High in lysine, they also contain tyrosine, a chemical needed to produce thyroid hormones.

- **Radishes:** An antiviral food that holds the magical sulfur that retards EBV with its smoke-screen effect. Help prevent and reduce thyroid cancer and remove radiation from the thyroid. When the thyroid gets depleted and beaten down from EBV, it gets hungry for trace minerals. Even when the land seems barren, radishes uptake over 30 trace minerals from the earth that are specifically beneficial for revitalizing and strengthening the thyroid. Radishes also help prevent thyroid atrophy.

- **Raw honey:** The best replenishing fuel there is to feed and revitalize the thyroid. The glucose and other nutrients in raw honey practically get mainlined into the thyroid to feed the gland. Medical science doesn't yet have its finger on the pulse of the symbiotic relationship between honey and the thyroid. An antiviral, too, that helps fight EBV with its zinc content.

- **Sesame seeds:** Strengthen the central nervous system while providing amino acids such as tyrosine and lysine in highly bioavailable trace forms that easily enter and uptake into the thyroid to improve the gland's function and suppress EBV.

- **Spinach:** Creates an alkaline environment in the body and provides highly absorbable micronutrients to the nervous system. Binds onto and removes the jelly-like viral waste matter in the liver that can contribute to mystery weight gain and mystery heart flutters. Especially good at rejuvenating skin and turning around conditions such as eczema and psoriasis.

- **Sprouts and microgreens:** High in zinc and selenium to strengthen the immune system against EBV, they also contain critical micronutrients for your thyroid and help reduce the growth of nodules.

- **Squash** (especially zucchini and spaghetti squash): Helps stabilize your thyroid and increase its production of thyroid hormones T4 and T3. Helps restore your liver and support its ability to convert thyroid hormones. Provides easily assimilable glucose for the brain and the rest of the nervous system to help heal inflamed nerves caused by EBV.

- **Sweet potatoes:** Help cleanse and detox the liver from EBV byproduct and toxins. Help nourish the skin and support the adrenal glands. Help reduce fibroids and cysts throughout the body caused by EBV, including the ovarian cysts that result in PCOS.

- **Thyme:** An incredible antiviral that's integral to cleaning up every thyroid disease. Its nutritional compounds get into the thyroid, killing off EBV there and allowing the thyroid to regain control of itself, while this valuable food also knocks down the viral load throughout the body, helping to relieve a multitude of symptoms.

- **Tomatoes:** Contain their own variety of vitamin C that's bioavailable to the lymphatic system and liver, supports the immune system to keep it strong against EBV, and prohibits the virus from traveling through the body with ease. This vitamin C is also a support to the thyroid's own immune system in the neck area. When growing, tomatoes absorb and collect the moonlight's frequency at night, just as the thyroid collects the sun's rays during the day (as you'll read about in Chapter 25, "Thyroid Healing Techniques"). This means that when consumed, tomatoes strengthen the thyroid's radio-like frequencies, helping to create balance and homeostasis with all of the body's organs and glands.

- **Turmeric:** Helps restore thyroid tissue, allowing the thyroid to regenerate and restore. Works on addressing viral issues throughout the body, acting as an anti-inflammatory as it knocks down EBV and reduces your viral load.

- **Watercress:** Helps stop the growth of EBV-caused scar tissue in the liver and thyroid. Pushes out old storage bins of pharmaceuticals such as thyroid medication from the liver, unburdening it from buildup so you can lose weight.

- **Wild blueberries:** Help restore the central nervous system and flush EBV neurotoxins out of the liver. Contain exceptionally powerful antioxidants that help repair your thyroid's tissue and reduce the growth of nodules. Help remove toxic heavy metals from the brain and liver. Ultimately, this all means that wild blueberries stop a shrinking brain and a shrinking thyroid. Not to be confused with their larger, cultivated cousins, wild blueberries can be found in the freezer section of many grocery stores.

stage of EBV, and it's great for dampening nodule growth.

- **L-lysine:** By inhibiting and reducing an EBV viral load, this amino acid acts as an anti-inflammatory to the entire nervous system, especially the central nervous system and the vagus and phrenic nerves, which get targeted by EBV's neurotoxins.

- **Chaga mushroom:** Kills off EBV, driving it out of the liver and thyroid. At the same time, stimulates the liver, elevating it out of stagnation and sluggishness, while awakening the thyroid, allowing it to improve function. Helps strengthen the adrenals. Also helps break down and dissolve EBV's biofilm byproduct that's behind so many cases of mystery heart palpitations.

- **5-MTHF (5-methyltetrahydrofolate):** Extremely helpful for supporting reproductive health that's been threatened by EBV, this supplement will be your ally in trying to come back from EBV-caused issues such as infertility, PCOS, and endometriosis. It also helps strengthen the endocrine and central nervous systems, promote methylation, and reduce homocysteine levels.

- **Barley grass juice extract powder:** Amazing for aiding in the elimination of mercury and other toxic heavy metals from the body. Holds specific alkaloids that help prevent the thyroid from atrophying while also blocking EBV

from feeding off its favorite foods, such as toxic heavy metals, inside the thyroid.

- **Monolaurin:** This antiviral breaks down an EBV viral load and reduces its cofactors such as strep.

- **Silver hydrosol:** Another potent antiviral, silver helps lower an EBV load, especially during the virus's chronic mono phase, when EBV is active in the bloodstream.

- **L-tyrosine:** This amino acid feeds healthy thyroid tissue even when the thyroid is under attack from EBV, so that the gland can continue with its production of thyroid hormones.

- **Ashwagandha:** While this herb does bolster the thyroid, the main reason to bring it into your life is to minimize adrenal surges that can feed EBV. By stabilizing the adrenal glands, ashwagandha helps prevent them from overproducing fear-based hormone blends that give fuel to EBV. (For a much more thorough understanding of the adrenal glands, see *Medical Medium*.)

- **Red marine algae:** This powerful antiviral helps remove heavy metals such as mercury from your system and reduces an EBV viral load.

- **Nettle leaf:** With vital micronutrients for the blood and central nervous system (particularly the brain), this top adaptogenic herb is also an anti-inflammatory for those organs infected with EBV. It's incredible for bringing you back to homeostasis—getting your body balanced again so everything functions better, including your lymphatic system, liver, and blood.

- **B-complex:** These are essential vitamins for the endocrine system, though their truly critical role is in supporting the central nervous system, which gets bombarded by EBV's neurotoxins.

- **Magnesium:** This homeostasis mineral is all about keeping thyroid hormone production in balance so that the thyroid neither under- nor overproduces hormones. It can also be helpful in reducing the neurological symptoms we looked at in Chapter 5.

- **EPA and DHA (eicosapentaenoic acid and docosahexaenoic acid):** These omega-3 fatty acids fortify the endocrine system and help strengthen the central nervous system so it's less susceptible to damage from the excessive amounts of adrenaline that can result from a thyroid condition, an overabundance of stress in your life, or both. Keep in mind EPA/DHA is only a fraction of brain health. Despite this trend that omegas are everything, the truth is that the majority of brain support comes from healthy carbohydrates like the foods in this chapter. Also, be sure to buy a plant-based (not fish-based) version.

- **Bladderwrack:** Another plant from the sea that provides easily assimilable trace minerals for the thyroid, as well as iodine to act as an EBV antiseptic so that viral cells will die off, ultimately enhancing the thyroid's function. Removes toxic heavy metals from the intestinal tract, which helps starve EBV.

- **Selenium:** Rather than killing off EBV, this supplement helps by strengthening thyroid tissue to protect it from scarring by the virus. It also boosts the overall immune system, strengthens and supports the central nervous system, and, via its support of the thyroid gland, helps stimulate production of the thyroid hormones T4 and T3.

- **Curcumin:** By strengthening the body's central and peripheral nervous systems, this component of turmeric acts as an anti-inflammatory and reduces nerve swelling caused by EBV's neurotoxins.

- **Chromium:** Supportive for the adrenals, thyroid, and the rest of the endocrine system, this supplement also aids pancreas and liver function to help stabilize your system as it fights EBV.

- **Vitamin D$_3$:** Supplementing with this vitamin helps stabilize the immune system and prevent it from overreacting to invaders such as EBV. Don't overdo it, though. As I explain in *Medical Medium Life-Changing Foods*, megadoses of vitamin D are not productive.

- **Manganese:** A critical supplement for production of the thyroid what will work for you and guide yourself back on course with compassion.

With each new month, check in with yourself. Had you planned to amp up to Choice C, and you're not feeling ready? Had you intended to dial it back to Choice A, and you feel too good to stop? In both these cases, try repeating whichever month feels comfortable instead. When you reach the next month, see where you stand and reassess.

At the end of the 90 days, you may find that you feel inspired to keep going. I've heard from many people who set out on the 28-Day Healing Cleanse from *Medical Medium* and felt so great at the end of the four weeks, with all of their symptoms gone, that they wanted to continue. You have that option here, too. Feel free to turn it into the 120-Day Thyroid Rehab or the 365-Day Thyroid Rehab.

Don't be discouraged if it takes you a year or a year and a half to heal. Don't lose faith. Healing will begin immediately, even if your symptoms are still with you for a while. Recovery simply takes time if the thyroid virus has been active in your system for many years, or if it's a variety that has caused you particularly difficult symptoms. Know that I see you. Hang in there. The reward—getting your life back—is worth it.

If you're someone who cleanses fast and gets overwhelmed with detox symptoms, you don't have to go all in with any choice at the beginning. Instead, select one bullet point from Choice A to add to your life, follow the list of what to avoid, and see how those two steps go for a while. When you're ready, you can work your way up to incorporating the other bullet points.

Like I said, it's all about what you need in *your* life, not some arbitrary belief system or trend.

One thing the Thyroid Rehab is definitely not about is deprivation or going hungry. I often find that when people try any sort of cleanse,

they tend to go into diet mode and undereat. Don't let this be you! Not only will this make it harder to sustain the changes, you'll also strain your adrenals by starving yourself. For optimal adrenal support as you heal, try to eat every hour and a half to two hours. Snacking is key.

Remember: This is about starving the virus, not starving you. It's about filling you up with delicious nutrition to fortify your thyroid and the rest of your body so you can shake off your symptoms and reclaim your life. Especially with Choice C, when you'll make the most changes that may be outside of your normal routine, remember to eat to feel full, supplement meals with snacks, and plan ahead so that you aren't stranded for food on trips or at social gatherings

For emotional support as you crowd out some of the unproductive foods during this cleanse, you may find it helpful to see the chapter "Food for the Soul" in *Medical Medium Life-Changing Foods*. And if you need help coming up with vibrant, delicious, healing meals, see the next chapter, "Thyroid Healing Recipes," for dozens of options, plus check out the 50 recipes in *Life-Changing Foods*.

As you read through each choice in the pages to come, the simplicity of the months' plans may strike you. Don't let their simplicity fool you. Sometimes it's the simplest of measures that people write off as too straightforward to make a difference in how they feel, when it's really just the opposite. Celery juice, for example, is a cornerstone of each choice—straight, unadulterated celery juice with no superfood boosters or powders mixed in. That's because celery juice on its own is an undiscovered superfood with a complex nutritional makeup. Only on its own can celery juice work its wonders. Alkalizing, enzyme-rich, electrolyte-enhancing, DNA-repairing, blood sugar–balancing, antiseptic, and more, this tonic is a "simple" step toward health that's not to be overlooked.

And so it goes for the rest of these steps. Most people who have struggled with symptoms for a long time and tried many different healing modalities have become sensitive. Their digestive systems are sensitive, their central nervous systems are sensitive—their whole bodies are sensitive. The techniques in this chapter are the best ones to take care of both these sensitive individuals and those with more robust constitutions. When taken seriously and applied properly, these techniques hold great power.

Now get ready to enter a new phase in life: healing, becoming, rebirth. May the next 90 days be ones of joy and transformation.

CHOICE A:
LIVER, LYMPHATIC,
AND GUT RELEASE MONTH

What to Add

The following tonics are ones to add to your normal life, working them in around meals and snacks. *You're not meant to get through each day on these liquids alone.* Make sure you fuel yourself with enough food in between so that you don't go hungry. Also keep in mind that whatever type of eating philosophy you subscribe to, you'll want to make sure that some of the healing foods and supplements from the previous chapter are part of your daily routine for the best chance of healing quickly and efficiently.

- Every morning, drink roughly **16 ounces of celery juice** on an empty stomach. (Make sure it's fresh, plain celery juice, with no other ingredients. For instructions on how

to make it, see the next chapter. If you're sensitive and 16 ounces is too much, start with a smaller amount and work your way up. Celery juice is a medicinal, not a caloric drink, so you'll still need breakfast afterward to power you through the morning. Simply wait at least 15 minutes after drinking your celery juice before consuming anything else.)

- Sip roughly **16 ounces of lemon or lime water** at midday or in early afternoon. (Squeeze the juice from one half of a lemon or lime per 16 ounces of water.)

- Sip roughly **16 ounces of lemon or lime water** in late afternoon.

- Every evening, drink roughly **16 ounces of aloe water or cucumber juice**. (For guidelines on making fresh aloe water, see the next chapter. If you opt for cucumber juice, enjoy it either plain or juiced with some optional parsley or cilantro. If you're traveling and it's not possible to make aloe water or cucumber juice, try to sip an extra lemon water at night instead.)

What to Avoid

- Take out the unproductive foods from Chapter 21, "Common Misconceptions and What to Avoid": eggs, dairy (including milk, cream, yogurt, cheese, kefir, and ghee), gluten, canola, corn, soy, and pork.

How You're Healing

This month, you'll get all of the healing benefits of the Liver, Lymphatic, and Gut Release Month, you'll add in ginger's antispasmodic and antiviral support, plus you'll get to extract those toxic heavy metals from your body that are some of EBV's favorite fuels.

When consumed within 24 hours of each other, barley grass juice extract powder, spirulina, cilantro, wild blueberries, and Atlantic dulse provide the most effective method on the planet of removing heavy metals. (For an extra boost, add burdock to the mix.) These foods each have their singular strengths, performing slightly different roles in the detoxification process. During the removal process, metals can get "dropped" or dispersed back into the organs, at which point another member of the team will swoop in, grab the metal, and continue the journey toward the finish line. I call this "pass the football." On its own, each individual player isn't 100 percent effective; as a team, they are your anti–heavy metal secret weapon!

If you've tried other heavy metal detox approaches before and been dissatisfied with the process, keep in mind that this "pass the football" approach is different. With other heavy metal detox techniques, metals get dropped along the way in your system or redistributed, and this may give you pesky symptoms. The heavy metal detox in this month truly is different—it's designed for the most sensitive of people, with zero side effects, because the combination of foods grabs onto the metals and removes them from your body.

Plus, the foods give something back to you. In addition to helping to draw metals out of the body, all of these powerful foods leave behind vital nutrients for repairing heavy metal damage. When toxic heavy metals spend time in your organs and other areas of your body, they create small, corroded, empty cavities—which the nutrients in these food fill in, fortify, and restore.

If you get each of these foods into your diet every day—the heavy metal detox smoothie is a fast, easy, tasty way to do it—you'll give your body profound assistance in fighting off EBV so your thyroid can resurrect itself. Without heavy metals around, EBV can't thrive and proliferate, and the production of neurotoxins drastically decreases. Remember, when EBV feeds off of heavy metals such as toxic copper, arsenic, cadmium, lead, nickel, mercury, aluminum, steels, and alloys, the neurotoxins that it excretes are full of those metals and therefore particularly toxic, responsible for so many of the symptoms we looked at in Chapter 5, "Your Symptoms and Conditions—Explained." Taking heavy metals out of the equation is the best way to halt the development of those devastating neurological symptoms.

Keep in mind that many people have toxic heavy metals buried in the body, sometimes deep inside the organs and glands (including the thyroid), connective tissue, or even bones. It can take some time to draw them all out, so be patient and try to adopt the heavy metal detox portion of this month for as long as you can to extract the layers of these metals that are embedded within the body.

CHOICE C:
THYROID VIRUS CLEANSE MONTH

What to Add

As in the other months, the following items are ones to add to your normal life, working them in around meals and snacks. Though the smoothie can count as one meal or snack, and a full bowl of antiviral broth with its veggies can be filling enough to form the basis of another meal, *you're not meant to get through each day on these items alone.* Make sure you fuel yourself with enough other food so that you don't go hungry. Also keep in mind that whatever type of eating philosophy you subscribe to, you'll want to make sure that some of the healing foods and supplements from the previous chapter are part of your daily routine for the best chance of healing quickly and efficiently.

- Every morning, drink roughly **16 ounces of celery juice** on an empty stomach. (Make sure it's fresh, plain celery juice, with no other ingredients. For instructions on how to make it, see the next chapter. If you're sensitive and 16 ounces is too much, start with a smaller amount and work your way up. Celery juice is a medicinal, not a caloric drink, so you'll still need breakfast afterward to power you through the morning. Simply wait at least 15 minutes after drinking your celery juice before consuming anything else.)

- Every day, drink the **thyroid healing smoothie**. (See the recipe in the next chapter. This smoothie is a great option for breakfast. If you don't like it as a blended drink, consume the smoothie ingredients separately over the course of the day.)

- Sip roughly **16 ounces of lemon or lime water** at midday or in early afternoon. (Squeeze the juice from one half of a lemon or lime per 16 ounces of water.)

- Sip one cup **of ginger water** at any point in the day. (For instructions on making fresh ginger water, see the next chapter. If you're traveling and can't make it fresh, pack a dried tea bag to make ginger tea instead.)

- Sip one cup of **thyroid healing tea** at any point in the day. (See the recipe in the next chapter.)

- At any point during the day or evening, sip a minimum of **one cup of thyroid healing broth**. (See the recipe in the next chapter. If you'd like instead, enjoy it as the broth plus its chunky vegetables, or blend both together for a puréed soup.)

- Every evening, drink at least **16 ounces of thyroid healing juice**. (See recipe in the next chapter. If needed, you can drink the juice at another time of day.)

What to Avoid

- Take out the unproductive foods from Chapter 21, "Common Misconceptions and What to Avoid": eggs, dairy (including milk, cream, yogurt, cheese, kefir, and ghee), gluten, canola, corn, soy, and pork.

- Skip tuna, swordfish, and bass this month, too.

- Lower your fat intake by a minimum of 25 percent. If you eat animal proteins, this will probably mean cutting back on your portions of steak, hamburgers, chicken breasts, and the like. While in the process of getting rid of the thyroid virus, maybe even consider eating only one portion of animal protein a day. (This doesn't mean eliminating animal proteins altogether.) And if you're plant-based or vegan, you'll want to lower your consumption of oils, seeds, and nuts. You might have noticed that coconut, seeds, and nuts are listed as healing foods in the previous chapter. Because of their special benefits, they belong there. What's important is making sure that these don't dominate your diet while you're healing. I've seen some vegetarians and vegans base every meal and snack around these foods. Even though they're healthy fats, you want to make sure you're leaving room for other healing foods.

How You're Healing

If Choice A is the starter model and Choice B is the upgrade, then Choice C is the deluxe version of the Thyroid Rehab, aimed at taming the thyroid virus when smaller measures won't do. You'll take it all to the next level with thyroid healing tea, mineral-rich thyroid healing broth, thyroid healing juice, and lower fat.

Because you're focused on cleansing the virus this month, you'll tone down the heavy metal detox, while still incorporating chelation foods such as Atlantic dulse, parsley, kelp, and cilantro. If you're up for it, you're still more than welcome to enjoy the heavy metal detox smoothie this month, or to incorporate its ingredients into your meals every day. No matter which direction you go, you'll want to make sure that you're still eating wild blueberries.

After reading about the benefits of thyme, fennel seed, and lemon balm in the previous chapter, you know just how important these are in fighting the thyroid virus—which is why you'll love bringing the thyroid healing tea into your life. By adding the thyroid healing broth to your daily routine, too, you'll be delivering precious virus-fighting nutrients to your body in a form that's easy to digest and assimilate. With the thyroid healing juice, you'll end the day well hydrated, with vital anti-inflammatory nutrition so your body has the resources it needs to go after the thyroid virus and repair any damage it's done.

And why low fat? Because you want to support your body in optimum detox. As we looked at in "Common Misconceptions and What to Avoid," high fats in the bloodstream lower oxygen in the bloodstream, and oxygen is critical for fighting EBV. The higher the level of fat you have in your system, the less oxygen you have to protect you from the thyroid virus. (Oxygenation is on your side, and not to be confused with oxidation, which EBV creates a tremendous amount of during its fourth stage. Oxidation is a chemical reaction of the body's organ tissue with an invader such as EBV. It's there to retard oxygen; it's the process that leads to aging—which is why we eat antioxidants to fight oxidation. Oxygenation, on the other hand, is when your blood has the oxygen it needs to fight pathogens such as EBV.)

Fat thickens the blood and slows down detoxification, hampering the rate at which toxins such as heavy metals can leave your body. This may sound surprising, because the trend goes in the opposite direction, saying to eat lots of protein and fat. That trend has been useful—I know that many of you reading this have gone on high-fat diets that eliminated processed foods, and you've seen results. I'm proud of you. You did your body good by getting back to the basics of whole foods.

Now, if you're still dealing with a weight condition, thyroid condition, liver condition, or other thyroid virus symptoms, it's time to thin out your blood so you can heal. When you're still dealing with thyroid virus symptoms, then the higher your fat intake, the better the virus is shielded from leaving your body. Whether you're high-protein, plant-based, vegan, or otherwise, if you're trying to get rid of the thyroid virus, then eating a diet high in fat, no matter how healthy those fats are, gives your liver extra work, which is the opposite of what you want when it's already doing so much for you by processing out EBV and other toxins from your system.

In order to flush out EBV debris, revive the thyroid, remove heavy metals, and kill off the thyroid virus, it's important to lower your fat intake. This thins out the blood, allowing viral waste product, the virus itself, bacteria, and those toxic heavy metals to leave your bloodstream, find their way to the kidneys and intestinal tract, and be eliminated. This doesn't mean you should cut out fats entirely, only that you'll get the best results by cutting *back*.

What Choice C translates to is a full-body restorative, giving your immune system incredible support to get rid of the virus while your thyroid gets its best chance at revival. If you'd like to supercharge this month, you can also opt to eat only living foods (raw fruits and vegetables) until dinnertime, or you can combine the Thyroid Virus Cleanse suggestions with the guidelines from the 28-Day Healing Cleanse in *Medical Medium*.

To fill yourself up when you're eating lower fat and avoiding foods such as wheat and soy, you'll find that fruit is your best resource. With its healthy carbohydrates and essential brain- and liver-fueling glucose that's bonded to vital phytochemicals, fruit is nature's disease-fighting gift to you. Misinformation out there might have kept you from fruit for years. It's time to leave that baggage behind.

Most fruit fear stems from the belief that fruit is too high in sugar—which completely disregards the reality that the sugar in fruit is not the same as refined table sugar or high-fructose corn syrup. Fruit digests so easily that its sugar leaves your stomach within minutes after you've eaten it—it doesn't even reach your intestinal tract, so contrary to health fads that say otherwise, it doesn't breed issues like *Candida*. Fruit is made up of so much: pulp, fiber, water, vitamins, minerals . . . all of which are wonderfully beneficial to your healing process. If you'd like to know more about fruit myth-busting, I get into the topic in much more depth in the chapter "Fruit Fear" in my first book, *Medical Medium*. For now, know that fruit, especially when combined with leafy greens, is one of the most sustaining allies you'll ever have.

In the next chapter, you'll find no shortage of ideas for how to make fruits—and other healing foods—into delicious, nourishing dishes to support you during your individualized Thyroid Rehab.

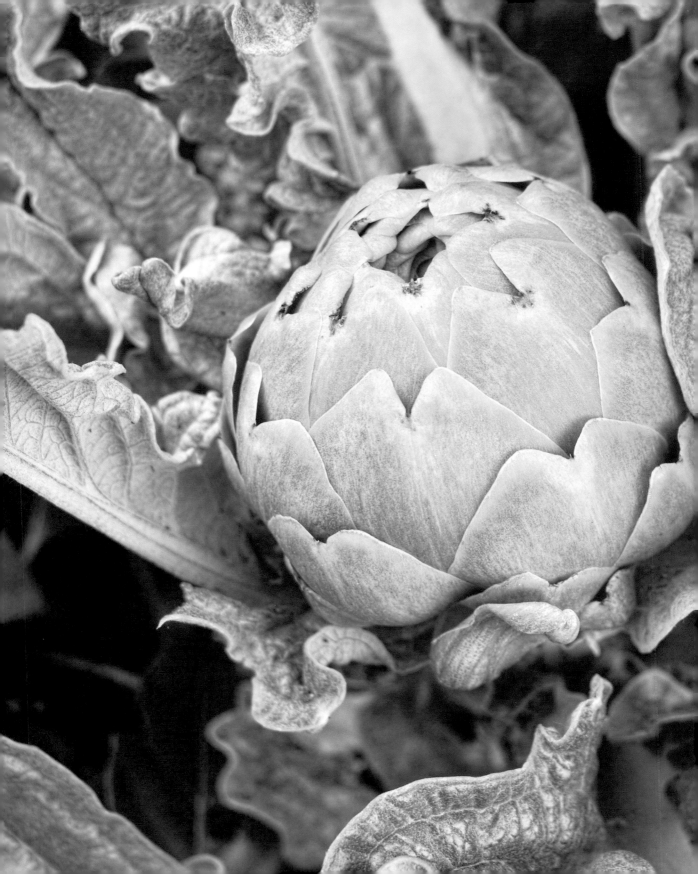

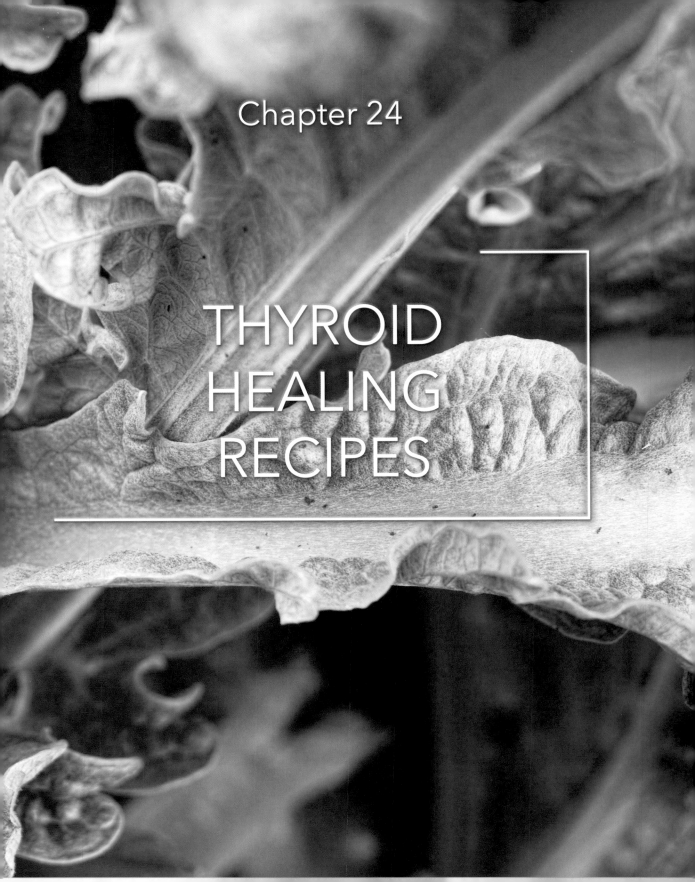

Chapter 24

THYROID
HEALING
RECIPES

THYROID HEALING JUICE

Makes 1 serving

This juice is made entirely of ingredients that support thyroid health. The best part is that it's easy to customize according to your tastes. Feel free to substitute cucumbers in place of the celery or parsley in place of the cilantro. In any case, you will be getting a big dose of powerful thyroid support!

1 bunch celery

2 apples, sliced

1 bunch cilantro

2 to 4 inches fresh ginger

Run all the ingredients through the juicer. Drink the juice immediately on an empty stomach for best results.

Alternatively, roughly chop the celery and apples. Add all of the ingredients to a high-speed blender. Blend the ingredients until smooth and then strain. Drink the resulting juice immediately.

TIPS

- As mentioned above, this juice can be customized to your taste preferences by substituting 2 cucumbers in place of the celery or 1 bunch of parsley in place of the cilantro.

- Depending on the juicer, more or less ginger will be needed. Adjust the amount according to your taste.

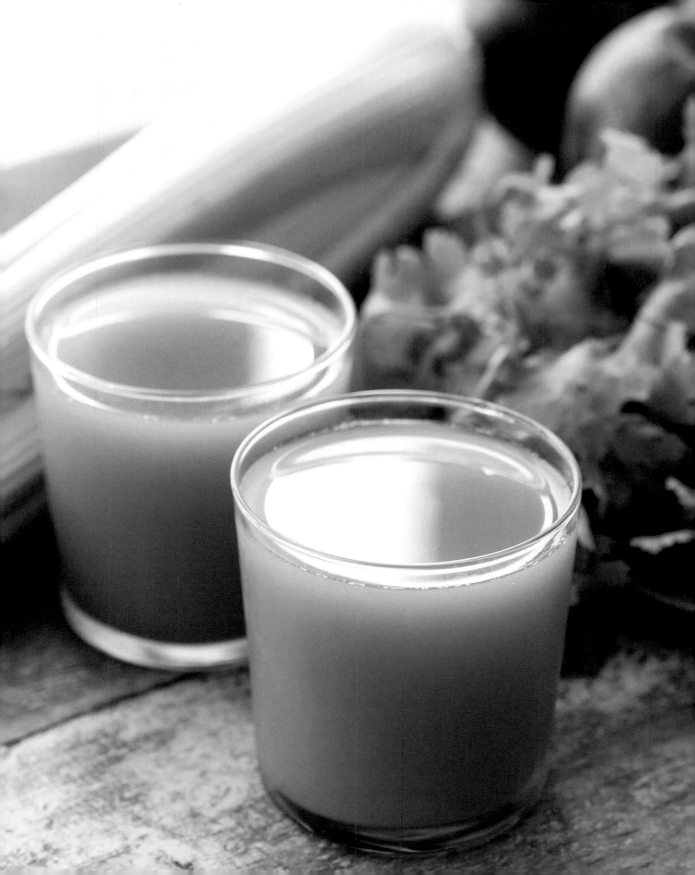

THYROID HEALING TEA

Makes 1 serving

Teas are a wonderful way to add some quiet to the busy rush of our days. This healing tea will do just as much for your spirit as for your thyroid and the rest of your body. As you drink, take a moment to pause and calm your heart and mind. What a miracle that such healing foods are available to us here on the earth!

2 cups water

1 teaspoon thyme

1 teaspoon fennel seed

1 teaspoon lemon balm

2 teaspoons raw honey
(optional)

Bring 2 cups of water to boil in a small saucepan. Add thyme, fennel seed, and lemon balm. Turn off the heat and allow the tea to steep for 15 minutes or more. Strain the tea and pour it into a mug. Stir in honey if desired and enjoy!

TIPS

- Store-bought tea bags can be used as well when loose tea is not available. Use one tea bag each of thyme, fennel seed, and lemon balm.

- Either fresh or dried thyme and lemon balm can be used.

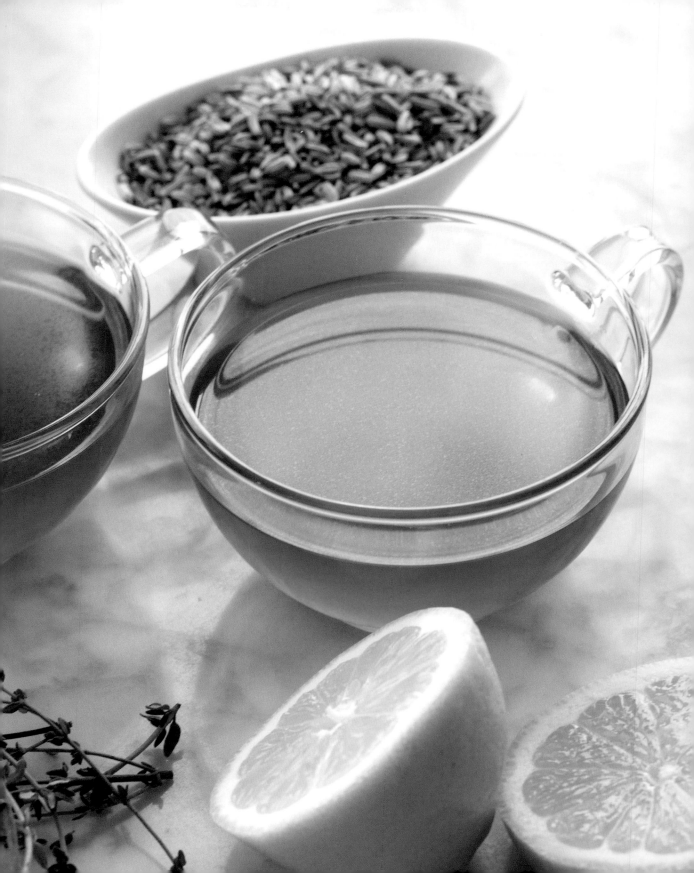

LEMON OR LIME WATER

Makes 1 serving

A tall glass of lemon or lime water is one of the very best tools for hydration and detoxification. On top of the healing benefits you read about in Chapter 22, lemons and limes activate drinking water, making it better able to latch onto toxins in your body and flush them out. Drinking this elixir, you'll feel like you are infusing every cell in your body with healing nectar!

½ lemon or lime

2 cups water

Squeeze the juice from half of a freshly cut lemon or lime into the water. Sip and enjoy!

TIP

- Lemons and limes travel well. When you're on the road and missing your kitchen, make sure to pack a few lemons and limes so you can enjoy this fresh tonic when you're far from home.

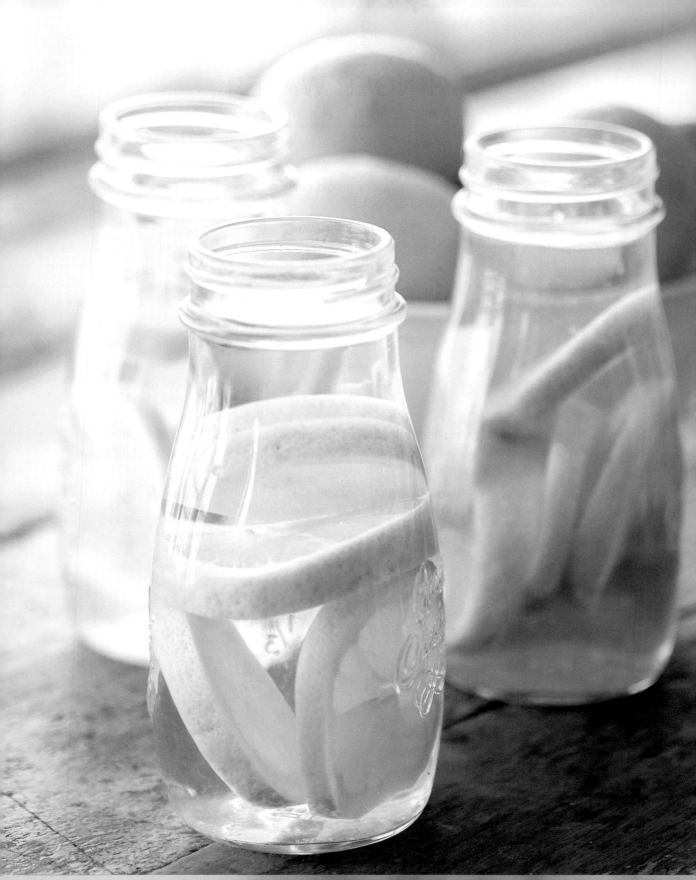

ALOE WATER

Makes 1 serving

While the taste of aloe may take some getting used to, it will be well worth the effort. As you drink your aloe water, think about all of the amazing benefits that your liver, your adrenals, and the rest of your body will reap from this amazing healing food.

2-inch piece of fresh aloe leaf

2 cups water

Scoop the gel from the inside of the fresh aloe leaf and place it into a blender alongside the water. Blend for 10 to 20 seconds until thoroughly combined. Drink immediately on an empty stomach for best results.

TIPS

- Fresh aloe leaves can be found in the produce section of many supermarkets.

- Save the remainder of the aloe leaf by wrapping the cut end in a damp towel or plastic wrap and storing in the refrigerator for up to 2 weeks.

- If you need to, you can also try blending aloe into a smoothie such as the Thyroid Healing Smoothie on page 192.

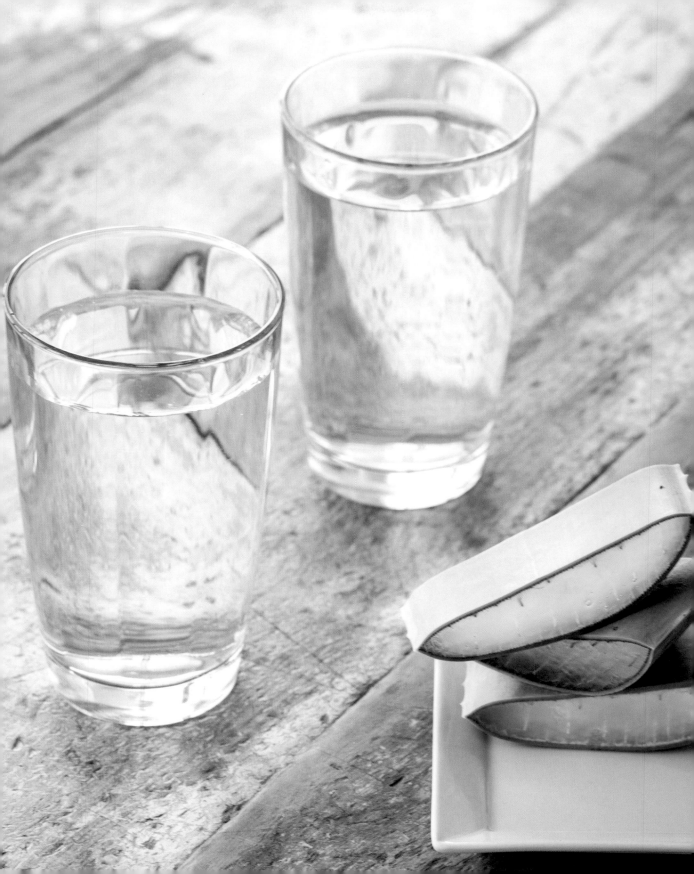

THYROID HEALING BROTH

Makes 1 to 4 servings

Sometimes it can feel challenging to stick to healthier ways of eating when all around you, others seem to indulge in less-than-productive foods. With this antiviral, mineral-rich broth—a cornerstone of the Thyroid Virus Cleanse Month featured in the previous chapter—you can give yourself a nourishing, comforting boost any time. If you'd like, keep a mug of it by your side all day, refilling as you desire.

2 sweet potatoes, cubed

2 celery stalks, diced

2 onions, diced

6 garlic cloves

1 inch turmeric root, peeled and minced

1 inch ginger, peeled and minced

1 cup finely chopped parsley

4 sprigs thyme

2 tablespoons Atlantic dulse flakes

1 tablespoon kelp powder

8 cups water

Place all the ingredients in a large pot. Bring the mixture to a boil, then reduce the heat to a low simmer for 1 hour. Strain and enjoy as a healing, restorative broth that can be sipped throughout the day.

TIPS

- This recipe may also be enjoyed as a chunky vegetable soup by leaving the vegetables in the broth.

- Alternatively, you can make a simple purée out of this recipe. Use an immersion blender to purée the vegetables until smooth or transfer them in small batches to a standing blender. Make sure to leave a vent for steam to escape through the top of the standing blender!

- You're welcome to make a large batch of this soup and freeze the leftovers to use throughout the week. Try freezing the broth in an ice cube tray for easy thawing later.

- If you'd like to make this soup a little more decadent to share with company, you can add a pinch of salt and a little splash of coconut oil into each individual bowl just before serving.

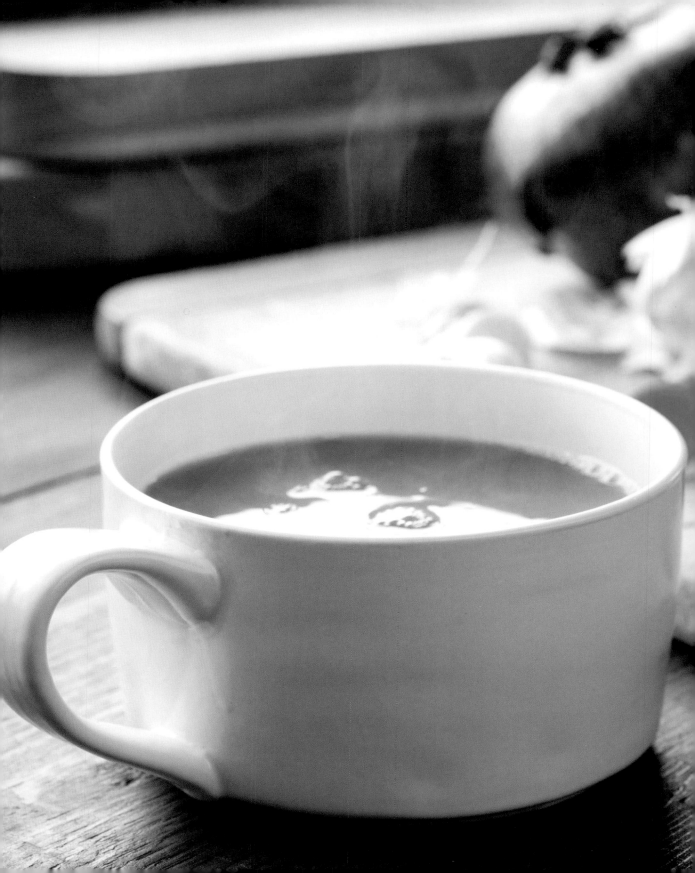

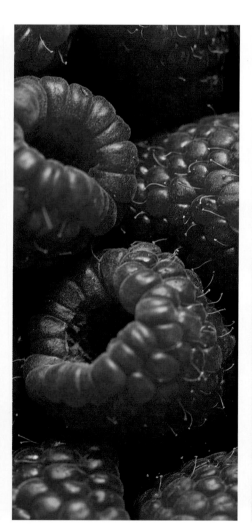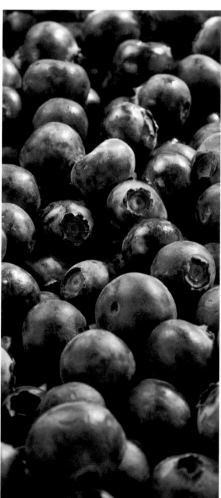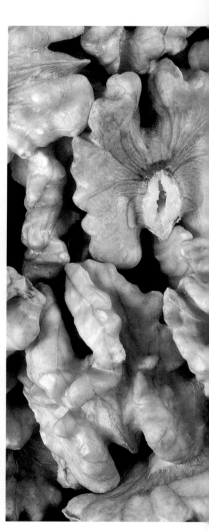

BREAKFAST

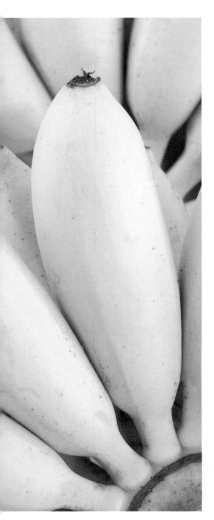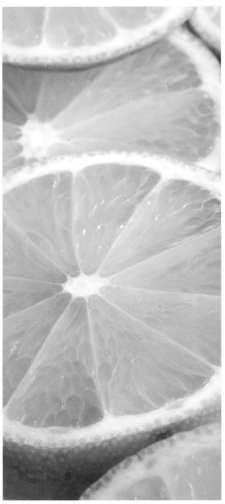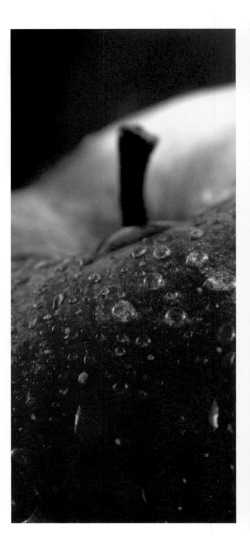

APPLE PORRIDGE
WITH CINNAMON AND RAISINS

Makes 1 serving

There's something so delightful about starting the day with a simple bowl of hearty goodness that's specifically geared to help you heal. In this version, skip the grains and load up on a bowl of fruit-based satisfaction.

3 apples, sliced

¼ teaspoon cinnamon

1 pinch vanilla bean powder

2 dates, pitted

1 teaspoon raw honey (optional)

½ lemon

¼ cup raisins

2 tablespoons walnuts (optional)

2 tablespoons shredded coconut (optional)

Combine the apples, cinnamon, vanilla bean powder, dates, honey, and the juice of the lemon in a food processor. Process all of the ingredients together until they are just combined. Pour the apple mixture into a bowl and stir in the raisins, walnuts, and shredded coconut if desired. Serve and enjoy!

TIP

- Feel free to get creative and figure out what toppings you like the most! Try different toppings on different days to get a variety of nutrients and flavors.

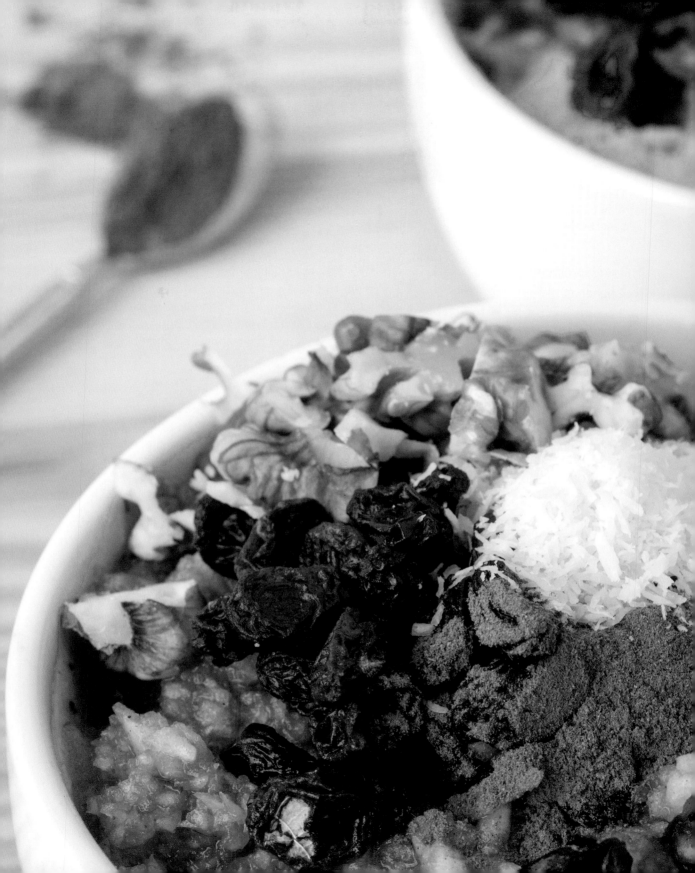

PAPAYA BERRY BOATS

Makes 2 servings

Delicious breakfasts don't have to be complicated! These papaya berry boats come together in minutes in a bright burst of color and flavor. They're perfect for a hydrating, satisfying breakfast that is easy to digest and will get your day started off right.

1 large Maradol papaya

2 bananas, sliced

3 cups mixed berries

1 lime (optional)

Slice the papaya in half lengthwise and scoop out the seeds. Place the two halves of the papaya on a plate with the cut sides facing up. Arrange the banana slices and the berries inside the center of each papaya half. Squeeze lime juice over the top of your papaya boats if desired and enjoy!

TIPS

- Maradol papayas are readily available in many supermarkets. If they're still green and unripe, look for ones with at least a hint of yellow-orange color in the skin. Left on the countertop, they will ripen until the skin gives when pressed, similar to a ripe avocado.

- If you're new to papaya's tropical flavor, lime juice is the perfect complement, which is why it's included as an optional ingredient in the list above. A simple squeeze of lime on papaya is a revelation worth experiencing.

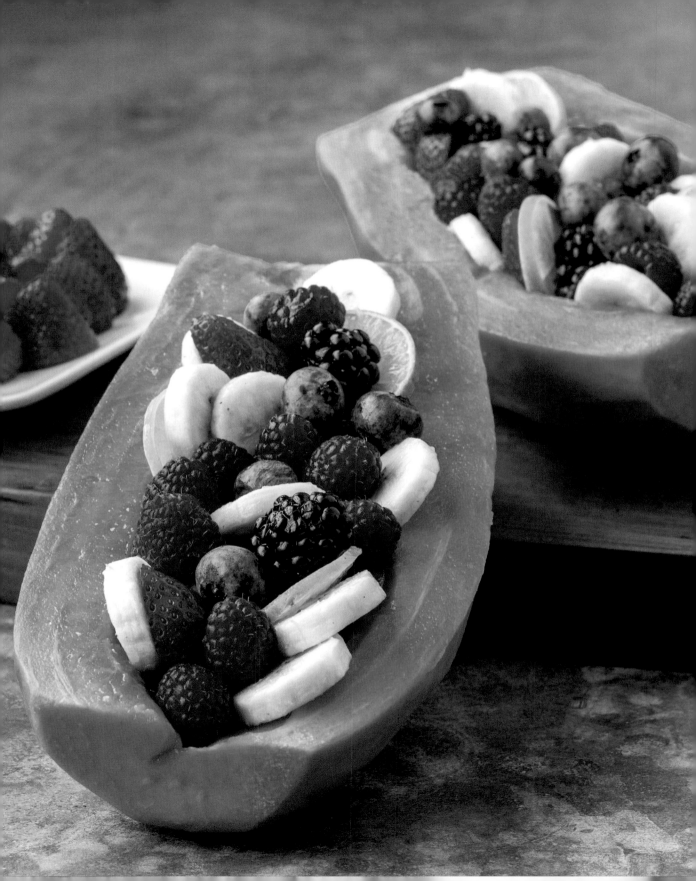

HEAVY METAL DETOX SMOOTHIE

This smoothie is a perfect and powerful combination of five key ingredients for detoxing heavy metals. Not only that—it tastes amazing!

2 bananas

2 cups wild blueberries

1 cup cilantro

1 teaspoon barley grass juice powder

1 teaspoon spirulina

1 tablespoon Atlantic dulse

1 orange

1 cup water

Combine the bananas, blueberries, cilantro, barley grass juice powder, spirulina, and dulse with the juice of one orange in a high-speed blender and blend until smooth. Add up to 1 cup of water if a thinner consistency is desired. Serve and enjoy!

TIPS

- If the barley grass juice powder and spirulina make the taste too strong for you, start with a small amount of each and work your way up.

- Keeping your kitchen stocked with ripe bananas is an art. Try asking your local grocer for an entire case of bananas (often available at a discount), then freeze a large batch when they reach peak ripeness. This way, you'll have frozen banans on hand for those days when you run out of fresh ones.

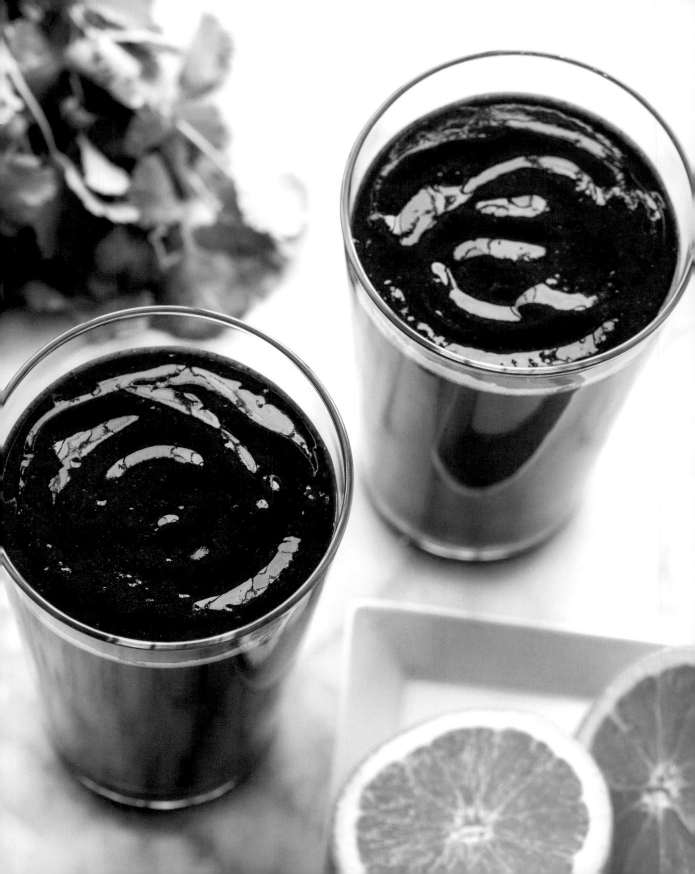

THYROID HEALING SMOOTHIE

Makes 1 serving

Smoothies are a great way to get a variety of healing ingredients in one go. You can customize this thyroid healing smoothie with whichever healing foods you'd like, rotating them throughout the week or month so that you get plenty of different nutrients and flavors.

2 cups mango (fresh or frozen)

1 banana

1 cup water

SUGGESTED ADDITIONS

2 cups spinach

½ cup arugula

1 teaspoon kelp powder

½ inch ginger, peeled

1 orange, juiced

½ cup cilantro

½ cup aloe vera gel

½ cup raspberries

Combine the mango and banana with 1 cup of water in a blender. Add any of the possible additions in assorted combinations. If you're feeling adventurous, go ahead and add them all! Blend until smooth. Serve and enjoy!

TIP

- For a change of pace, turn this into a light yet satisfying smoothie bowl, arranging sliced banana or peach, cubed mango or papaya, diced pear, pomegranate seeds, fresh or even frozen berries, raisins, or chopped dates, figs, or dried apricots on top.

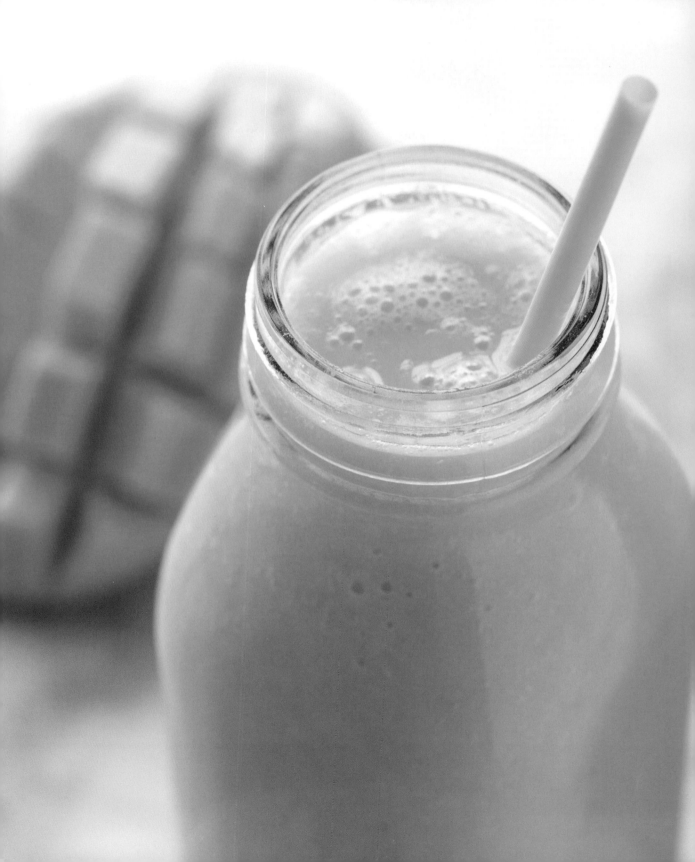

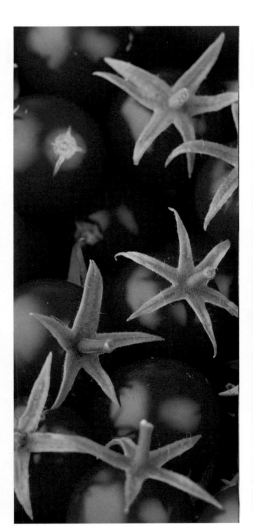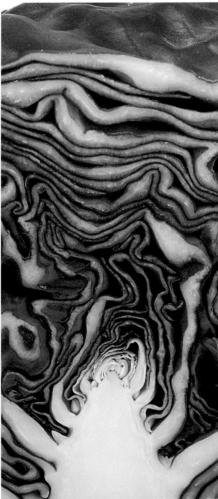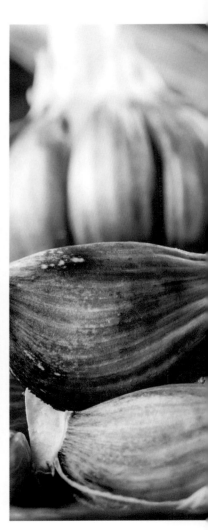

LUNCH

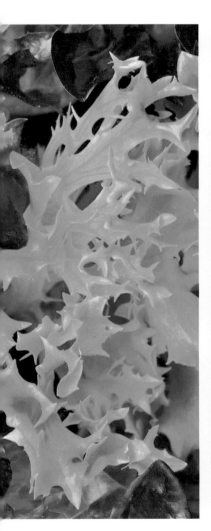
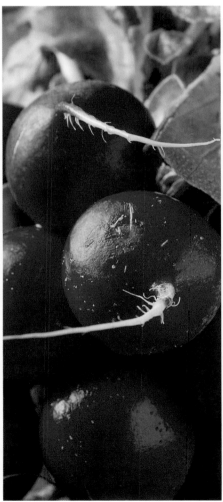
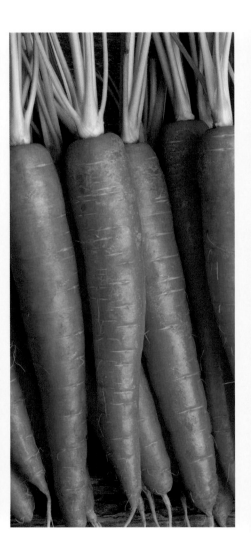

PESTO ZUCCHINI NOODLES

Makes 2 servings

These zucchini noodles are a bright and delicious way to enjoy so many beautiful ingredients together. The familiar flavors of pesto combine with sweet cherry tomatoes and mild noodles in a dish that is light, satisfying, and, simply put, wonderful!

3 medium zucchinis, peeled

2 cups loosely packed basil leaves

¼ cup hemp seeds

¼ cup walnuts

1 teaspoon olive oil (optional)

½ date

2 garlic cloves

¼ teaspoon sea salt

1 lemon

¼ cup water

2 cups cherry tomatoes

Turn your zucchinis into noodles using a spiralizer, peeler, or julienne peeler. Place these noodles into a large mixing bowl and set aside. Blend the basil leaves, hemp seeds, walnuts, olive oil, date, garlic cloves, sea salt, and juice of the lemon with the water until a smooth pesto forms. Pour the pesto over the zucchini noodles and toss until they are evenly coated. Divide the noodles between two bowls. Top with sliced cherry tomatoes. Serve and enjoy!

TIPS

- Kelp or cucumber noodles may be used in place of the zucchini noodles if desired.
- This dish is the perfect item to bring along to your next picnic in the park. Make a double batch that is big enough to share!

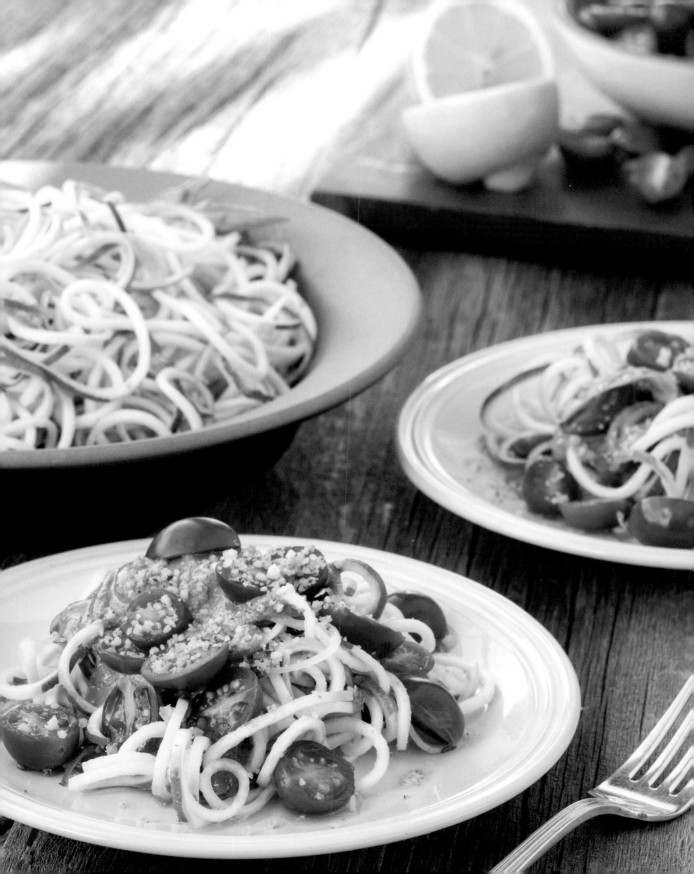

MASON JAR SALADS TWO WAYS

Makes 2 servings

One of the best ways to incorporate an abundance of healing foods into your diet is to prepare ahead of time. These two salads can be made in advance and stored in the fridge for up to 3 days. Keep them on hand for an easy grab and go meal anytime!

MIXED VEGETABLE SALAD WITH "RANCH" DRESSING

2 cups shredded red cabbage

2 cups shredded carrots

2 cups chopped asparagus

1 cup sliced radish

1 cup chopped fennel

1 cup chopped celery

1 cup chopped cilantro

½ cup chopped parsley

½ cup sliced scallion

1 lemon, halved

1 avocado, diced (optional)

8 cups spinach or arugula

RANCH DRESSING:

¼ cup Brazil nuts

¼ cup cashews

6-inch piece of celery

1 garlic clove

1 tablespoon dried parsley

1 tablespoon fresh dill

½ tablespoon garlic powder

¼ teaspoon celery seeds

¼ teaspoon sea salt

1 lemon

½ cup water

Layer all of the ingredients, except for the spinach or arugula, into two large (32-ounce) mason jars. Store the jars in the fridge for up to 3 days. Enjoy the mixed vegetables over a bed of leafy greens topped with "ranch" dressing.

Blend the Brazil nuts, cashews, celery, garlic clove, dried parsley, fresh dill, garlic powder, celery seeds, sea salt, and the juice of the lemon together until smooth. Slowly stream in ¼ to ½ cup of water, stopping when desired consistency is reached. Store the dressing in a small mason jar in the fridge for up to 3 days.

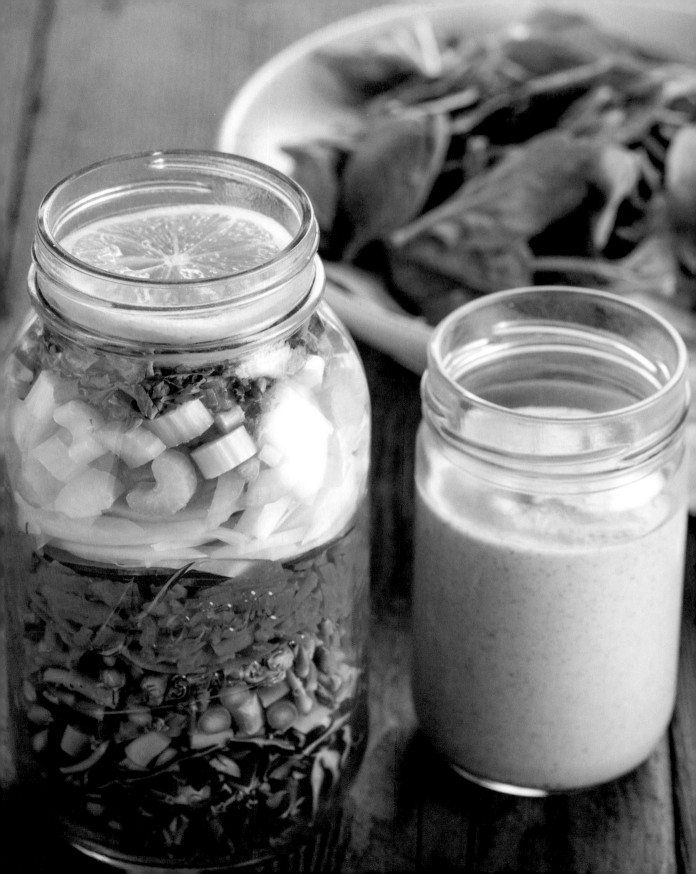

FRUIT SALAD WITH LEAFY GREENS

2 cups orange sections

2 cups raspberries

2 cups diced mango

2 cups diced cucumber

1 cup pomegranate seeds

1 cup chopped cilantro

½ cup chopped basil

1 lime

8 cups leafy greens

Layer all of the fruit into two large (32-ounce) mason jars. Slice the lime into wedges and layer them on the top of the jars' contents. Store the jars in the fridge for up to 3 days. Enjoy the fruit salad over a bed of mixed leafy greens with lime juice squeezed over the top.

TIPS

- If you don't have mason jars on hand, you can store these salads in any available container.

- If you're running out the door, grab a bag or box of pre-washed salad greens along with your salad jar, and you'll be ready to go. Don't let anything stop you from healing—you've got this!

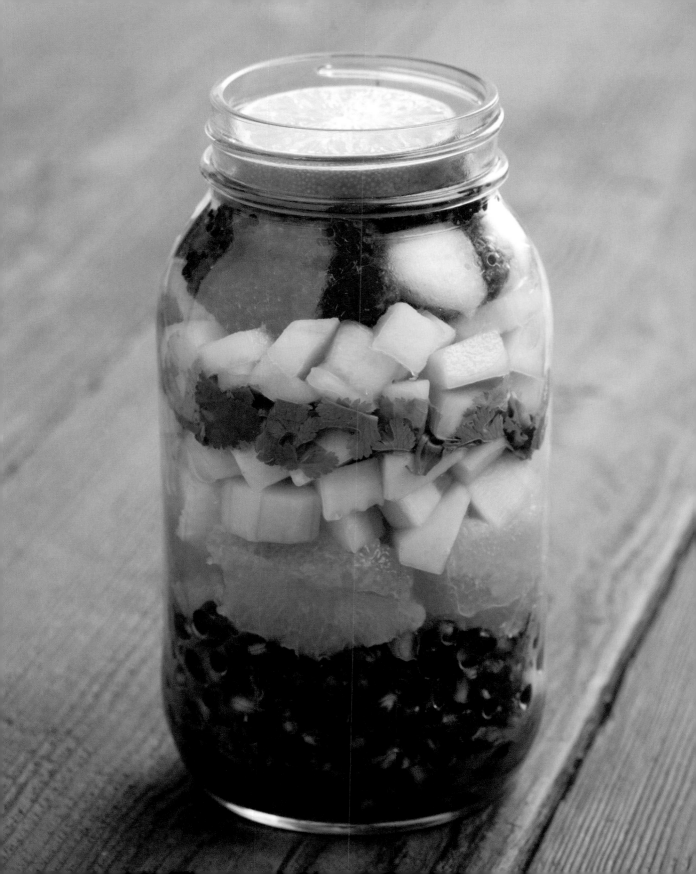

SPINACH SOUP

Makes 1 serving

One of the amazing things about incorporating more fruits and vegetables into our diet is the way that our taste buds change, and we begin to crave more and more of these fresh ingredients over time. When you find yourself yearning for leafy greens and the benefits they provide, this easy-to-make, richly flavored soup is a great way to incorporate them into your day in an easily digestible form. With all of the minerals the spinach provides, you'll also help curb any cravings for the foods you know don't serve your health right now.

1½ cups grape tomatoes

1 stalk celery

1 garlic clove

1 orange

4 cups baby spinach

2 basil leaves

½ avocado (optional)

Blend the tomatoes, celery, and garlic with the juice of 1 orange until smooth. Add the spinach by the handful until completely incorporated. Add the basil and the avocado (if desired), blending until creamy and smooth. Serve and enjoy immediately!

TIPS

- Cilantro may be used in place of the basil by substituting ¼ cup of cilantro leaves.

- If this soup doesn't have you singing "Hallelujah!" at the beginning of your journey, give it another try in a few weeks. As your palate begins to change, you may find that you wind up loving this soup so much that you make it a staple of your diet!

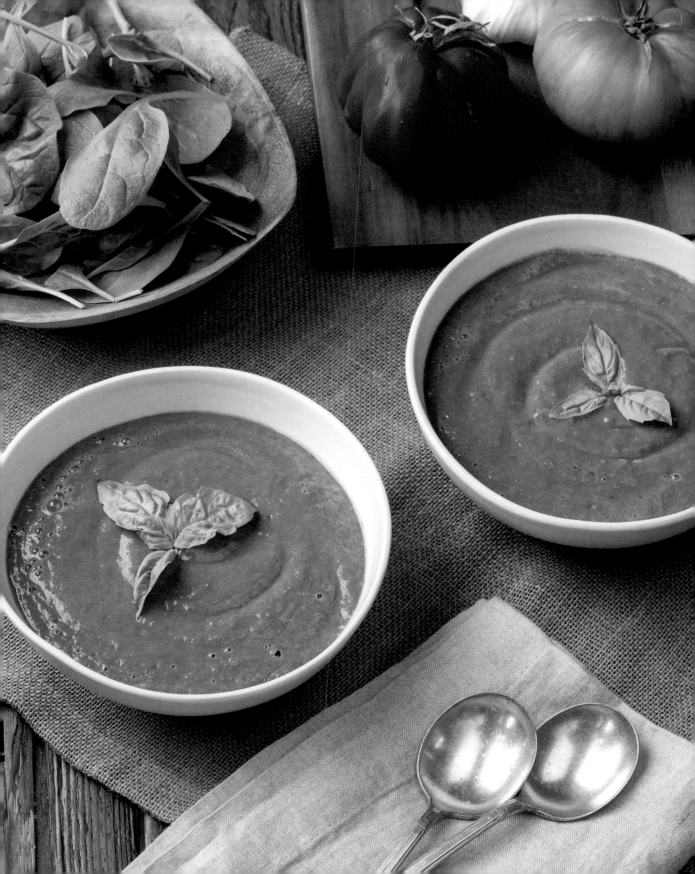

SUN-DRIED TOMATO ARTICHOKE DIP WITH VEGETABLE CRUDITÉS

Makes 2 servings

This creamy dip takes only seconds to prepare and combines bold flavors with comforting warmth. Sun-dried tomatoes, garlic, and parsley blend perfectly with tender artichoke hearts to create a dip that will have everyone coming back for more!

2 cups steamed artichoke hearts (see Tips)

¾ cup oil-free sun-dried tomatoes, soaked in hot water for 5 minutes

2 tablespoons raw tahini

1 cup loosely packed parsley

2 garlic cloves

1 lemon

¼ teaspoon sea salt

Vegetables of your choice for dipping (such as bell pepper, cucumber, cauliflower, radishes, asparagus)

Place the artichoke hearts, sun-dried tomatoes, tahini, parsley, garlic cloves, juice of the lemon, and sea salt into a food processor. Process the ingredients together until well combined. Serve the artichoke dip alongside any vegetables of your choice!

TIPS

- To prepare the artichoke hearts, follow the directions for steaming whole artichokes on page 212. Allow the artichokes to cool and then remove all of the tough green leaves until only the tender yellow leaves remain. Cut the artichoke in half and remove the choke (the silky white and purple leaves and the underlying filaments) completely by scooping it out with a spoon. Now your artichoke heart is ready to use.

- If raw tahini is unavailable, regular tahini may be used instead. Raw tahini has a milder flavor, and roasted tahini is more distinctive. Either will work well.

- Enjoy this dip with raw vegetables as described or with cooked vegetables of any kind. If you're feeling creative, you can even try stuffing it into a baked potato!

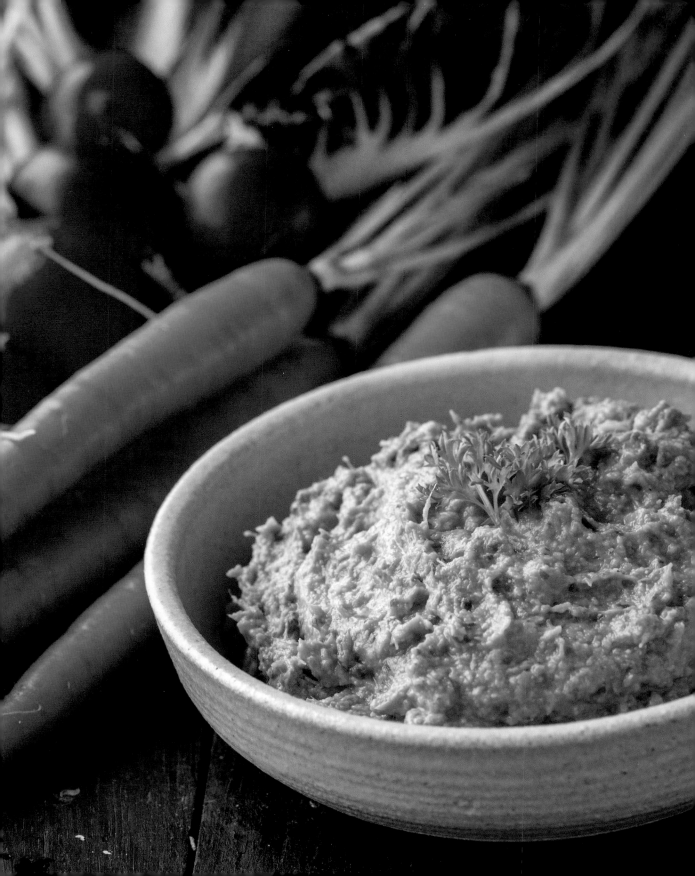

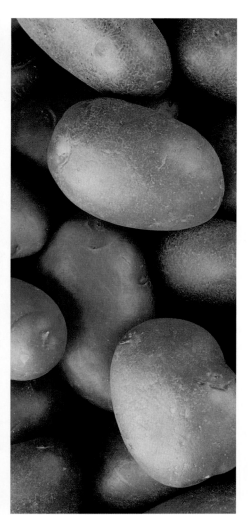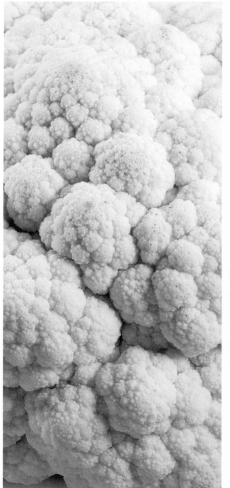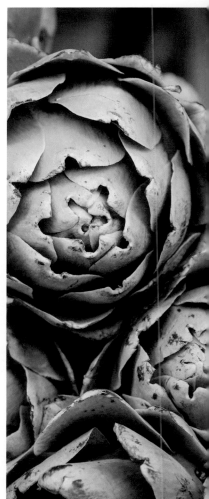

DINNER

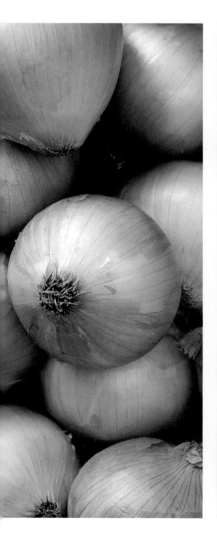
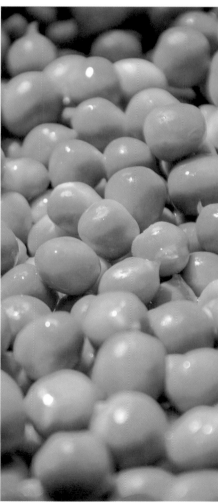
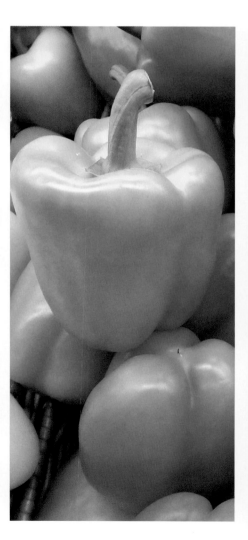

"NACHOS-STYLE" BAKED POTATOES

Makes 2 to 3 servings

While traditional nachos may involve chips, these soft and golden baked potato rounds leave nothing to be desired. Cooked perfectly in the oven until crispy on the outside and tender in the middle, then piled high with the familiar flavors of avocado, tomato, onion, and cilantro, these potatoes will disappear fast, so you may want to make a double batch. Make these potatoes extra indulgent by topping them with the Garlic Cashew Aioli on page 212!

6 medium potatoes

2 teaspoons coconut oil

½ teaspoon sea salt, divided

1 avocado, diced

1 cup diced tomato

1 cup diced onion

½ cup cilantro, chopped

½ jalapeño, minced (optional)

2 limes

¼ cup Garlic Cashew Aioli (optional, recipe on page 212)

Preheat the oven to 375°F. Peel and slice the potatoes into rounds that are ¼ inch to ½ inch thick. Toss them with the coconut oil and ¼ teaspoon of the sea salt. Arrange the potatoes on a baking tray lined with parchment paper. Leave space so that they are not touching or overlapping. Bake the potatoes for 20 minutes, flip, and then bake for 10 more minutes.

While the potatoes bake, combine the avocado, tomato, onion, cilantro, jalapeño, and the juice of both limes in a small mixing bowl. Arrange the potato slices in a pile on a serving plate. Top with the avocado salsa and drizzle the Garlic Cashew Aioli over the top if desired. Finish the nachos off with the remaining sea salt and enjoy!

TIPS

- Experiment with different varieties of potatoes for different nutrients, flavors, and textures.
- For a make-ahead trick, try peeling and slicing the potatoes in advance and storing them in a bowl of cold water in the fridge. They will keep well for up to three days this way; just change the water daily and enjoy having potatoes ready to go at a moment's notice.

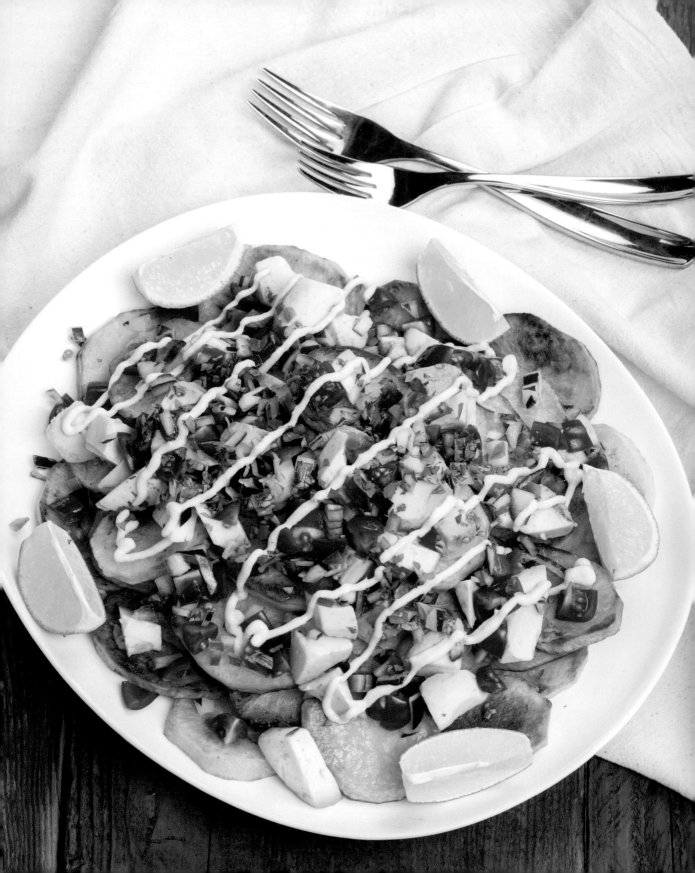

CAULIFLOWER "FRIED RICE"

Makes 2 to 3 servings

Juggling our healing journeys with the demands of busy schedules and the needs of our loved ones can be a challenge. This cauliflower "fried rice" may make your life a little easier with it's restaurant-quality flavor and fast prep time. It's a recipe that can be made cooked or raw, and it's easy to customize with your family's favorite vegetables and herbs.

1 medium cauliflower
(about 6 cups florets)

1 teaspoon coconut oil

½ red onion, diced

1 inch ginger, minced

3 garlic cloves, minced

1 large carrot, diced

1 red bell pepper, diced

2 stalks celery, diced

1 cup peas

1 teaspoon toasted sesame oil

2 tablespoons coconut aminos

½ teaspoon raw honey
(optional)

1 teaspoon sea salt

½ jalapeño (optional)

1 cup cilantro

¼ cup almonds, chopped
(optional)

2 teaspoons sesame seeds

1 lime

Cut cauliflower into florets and place into a food processor. Pulse until the cauliflower achieves a coarse rice texture. Use a nut milk bag or cheesecloth to wring extra moisture out of the "rice" and then set it aside.

Heat 1 teaspoon of coconut oil in a large pan and sauté the onion over medium-high heat until translucent and cooked through. Add water by the tablespoon as needed to prevent sticking. Place the ginger, garlic, carrot, bell pepper, celery, and peas in the pan with the red onion and continue to cook for 5 to 7 minutes until the vegetables begin to soften. Add the cauliflower rice, toasted sesame oil, coconut aminos, honey, and sea salt to the pan and stir well to combine. Continue to cook another 5 to 7 minutes until cauliflower rice is tender.

Serve the cauliflower "fried rice" topped with jalapeño (if desired) along with cilantro, chopped almonds, sesame seeds, and a generous squeeze of lime juice!

For raw cauliflower "fried rice": Follow the first step to make cauliflower rice, and place the rice into a large bowl along with the red onion, ginger, 1 clove of minced garlic, carrot, bell pepper, and celery. Stir the toasted sesame oil, coconut aminos, sea salt, and jalapeño into the cauliflower rice and marinate for at least 15 minutes. Serve topped with cilantro, chopped almonds, sesame seeds, and lime juice.

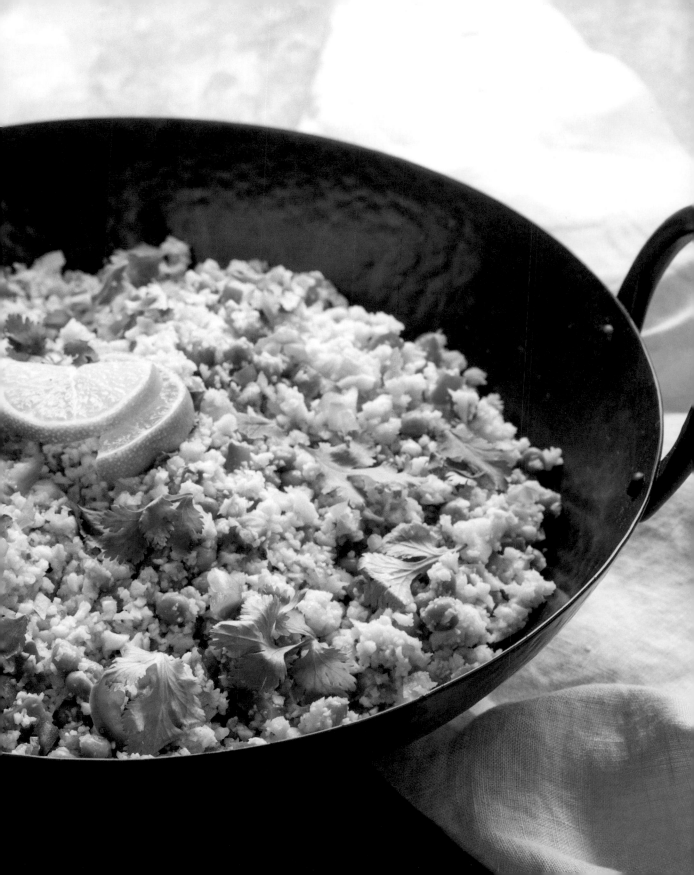

STEAMED ARTICHOKES
WITH GARLIC CASHEW AIOLI

Makes 2 servings

Steamed artichokes are delicious eaten on their own with a little lemon juice and sea salt—especially when you know about all of the healing benefits they bring to your thyroid. This recipe takes artichokes to another level, pairing them with a decadent garlic cashew aioli. It's an incredibly simple recipe to pull together and a great way to wow the guests at your next dinner gathering.

4 artichokes

1 cup cashews

2 tablespoons olive oil

3 garlic cloves

2 lemons

¼ teaspoon sea salt

½ to 1 cup water

Trim the artichokes by slicing ½ inch off of the tops and all but ½ inch off the stems. Trim any remaining leaves by ½ inch as well. Bring a pot of water to boil. Place the artichokes into a steamer basket inside the pot. Steam the artichokes for 30 to 40 minutes depending on size. They're done when one of the leaves pulls off easily and is tender.

Combine the cashews, olive oil, garlic, juice of two lemons, and sea salt in the blender with ½ cup of water. Blend until smooth for a thicker aioli. For a thinner consistency, continue to stream in another ½ cup of water while blending.

Serve the artichokes alongside the cashew aioli for dipping and top with any fresh herbs as desired!

TIP

- Save the extra aioli for use as a sauce over steamed potatoes or broccoli, as a topping for the "Nachos-Style" Baked Potatoes (recipe on page 208), or massaged into kale for a hearty salad.

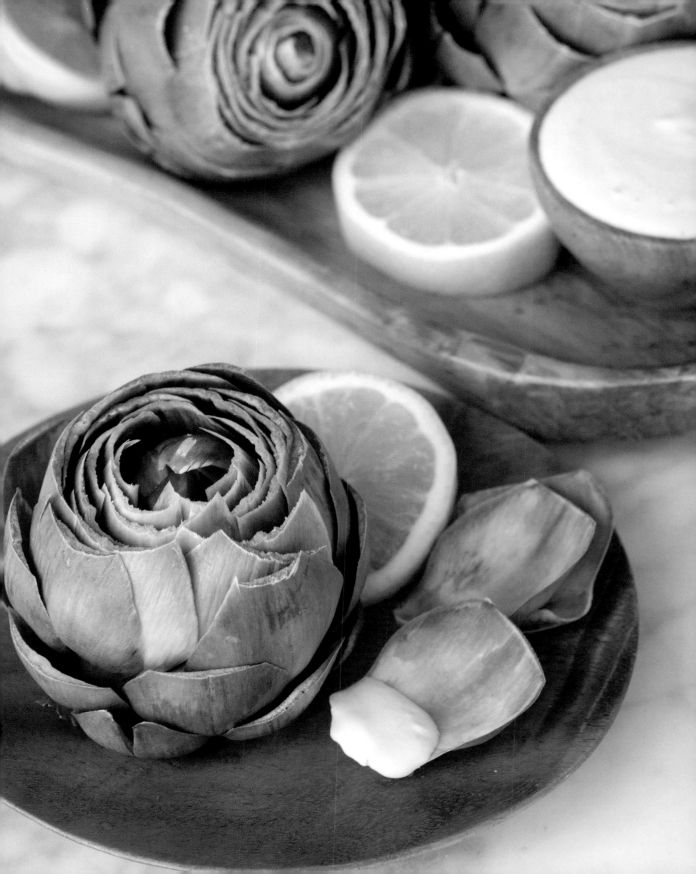

SPAGHETTI SQUASH "BOLOGNESE"

Spaghetti squash gets its name for a very good reason. The tender, yellow strands are so much like spaghetti, especially when you top them with a rich, savory tomato sauce and a sprinkle of Brazil Nut Basil "Parmesan." This dish will be an instant favorite with family and friends, so you might want to make a double batch. Freeze a batch of the sauce so that you always have some on hand when the urge for a big bowl of spaghetti strikes!

1 large spaghetti squash

2 cups diced red onion

4 garlic cloves, minced

2 cups cherry tomatoes

1 cup sliced mushrooms (optional)

1 teaspoon chili powder

1 teaspoon poultry seasoning

1 teaspoon garlic powder

¼ teaspoon curry powder

¼ teaspoon sea salt

½ cup sun-dried tomatoes, soaked 5 minutes in hot water

¼ cup Brazil Nut Basil "Parmesan" (see below)

BRAZIL NUT BASIL "PARMESAN"

¼ cup Brazil nuts

¼ teaspoon sea salt

¼ teaspoon dried basil

1 garlic clove

Preheat the oven to 400°F. Carefully slice the spaghetti squash in half and discard the seeds. Fill a baking tray with ½ inch of water and place the squash halves cut side down in the tray. Bake the squash for 30 to 40 minutes until one finger pressed gently into the exterior of the squash leaves an indentation. Remove the squash halves from the oven. When they are cool enough to handle, use a fork to scrape down the insides of the squash creating "spaghetti" strands. Divide the squash noodles between two bowls.

To make the "Bolognese," place the diced onion into a medium saucepan along with 2 tablespoons of water. Sauté the onion over medium-high heat until translucent and tender. Continue adding water by the tablespoon as needed to prevent sticking. Add the garlic, cherry tomatoes, mushrooms, chili powder, poultry seasoning, garlic powder, curry powder, sea salt, and sun-dried tomatoes to the saucepan and continue cooking, stirring frequently for 5 to 7 minutes, until the tomatoes soften. Using an immersion blender, blend the sauce ingredients together until combined but still chunky. Alternatively, transfer to a standing blender and pulse blend, making sure to leave the top ajar for steam to escape.

Serve the sauce over the top of the spaghetti squash noodles. Top with the Brazil Nut Basil "Parmesan" and enjoy!

Place the Brazil nuts, sea salt, basil, and garlic into the blender or food processor and pulse briefly until small crumbles form.

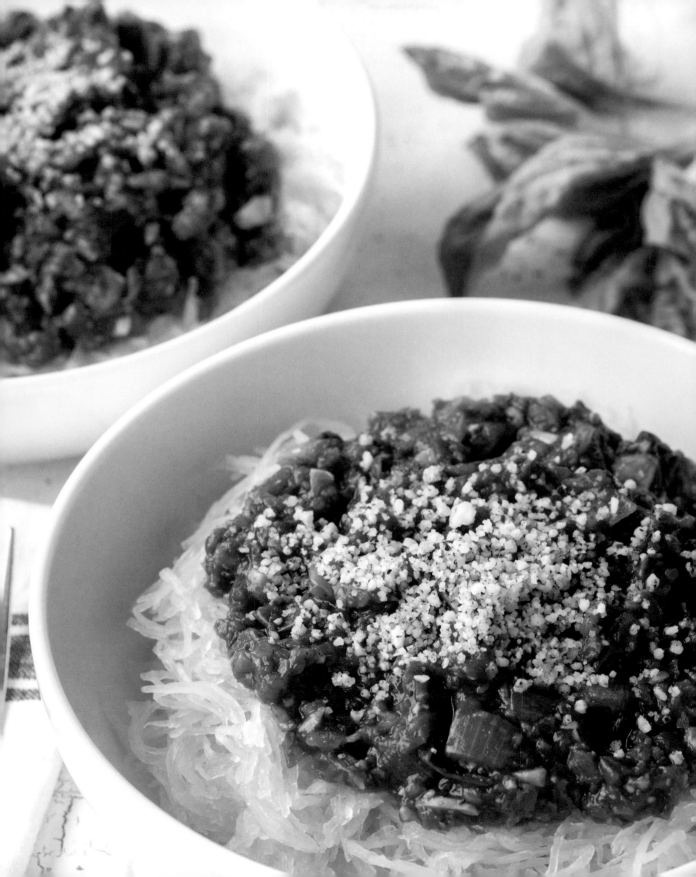

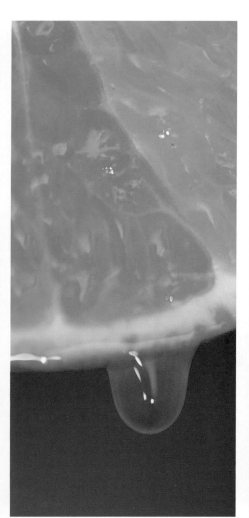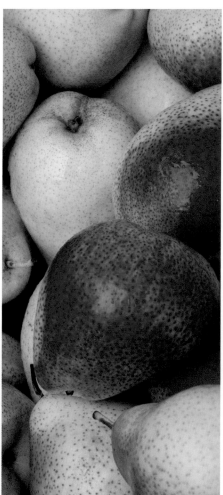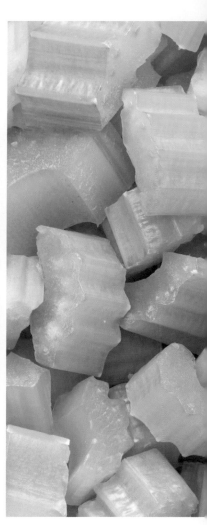

SNACKS

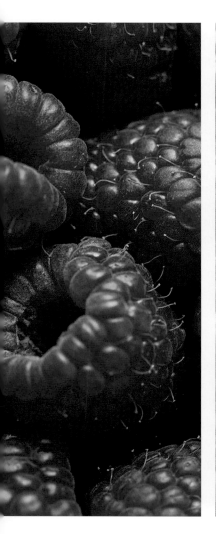
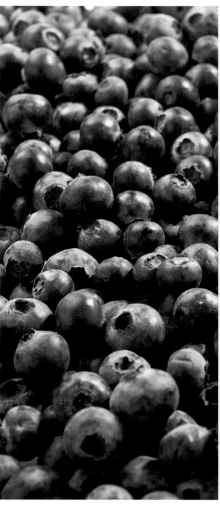
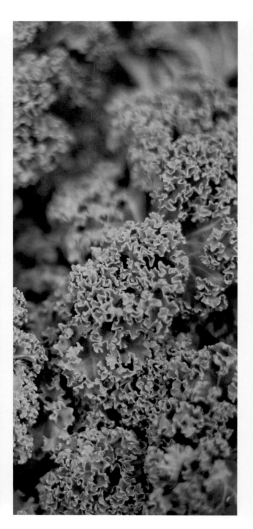

SWEET POTATO CHIPS AND GUACAMOLE

Chips get a bad reputation because many store-bought chips come loaded with preservatives and undesirable ingredients. It is possible to make delicious, clean chips right in the oven at home! The recipe below has a lot of spices for a bold, flavorful chip, though feel free to leave them all out. These chips are just as delicious with nothing more than a sprinkle of sea salt or dipped in this mouthwatering guacamole.

2 large sweet potatoes

¼ teaspoon sea salt

¼ teaspoon garlic powder

¼ teaspoon cumin

¼ teaspoon paprika

¼ teaspoon chili powder

¼ teaspoon cayenne (optional)

2 teaspoons coconut oil (optional)

GUACAMOLE

2 avocados

½ lemon

1 lime

1 small tomato, finely diced

¼ red onion, finely diced

½ cup cilantro, chopped

1 garlic clove, minced

¼ jalapeño, minced (optional)

¼ teaspoon sea salt (optional)

Preheat the oven to 250°F. Using a mandoline or knife, slice the sweet potatoes into very thin rounds, approximately ¹/₁₆-inch thick if possible and no thicker than ⅛ inch. Make sure they are even and thin, though not transparent. Bring a pot of water to boil. Place the sweet potato slices into the boiling water and return to a simmer over medium heat. After 5 minutes, remove the sweet potatoes and discard the water.

Combine the sea salt, garlic powder, cumin, paprika, chili powder, and cayenne in a small bowl. Lightly grease two baking trays with coconut oil. Arrange the sweet potato slices on the trays so that they are not overlapping. Brush the tops of the sweet potatoes lightly with more coconut oil. Sprinkle the spice mix generously over the top of the slices.

Bake the sweet potatoes for 25 minutes. Remove the trays from the oven and set the slices that are already crispy to one side. Return the trays to the oven for 5 more minutes and then check to remove the crispy chips again. If needed, bake the remaining slices 3 to 5 minutes more. Note that the chips might not appear crispy when first removed from the oven, though they should crisp up as they cool.

Serve sweet potato chips alongside guacamole, or enjoy them plain! For best results, serve shortly after making!

Mash the avocado together with the juice from the lemon and lime in a small bowl. Stir the tomato, onion, cilantro, garlic, jalapeño, and sea salt into the mashed avocado. Serve and enjoy with the sweet potato chips, alongside any cut-up vegetables of your choice, as a salad dressing, or even on top of cooked vegetables as desired.

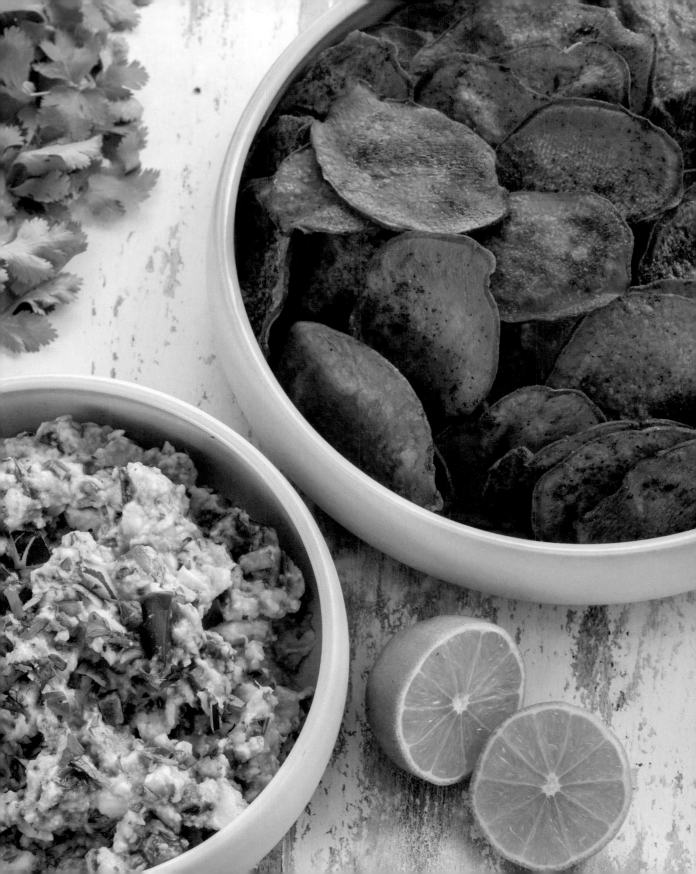

WILD BLUEBERRY BANANA ICE CREAM

This ice cream is everything you could want it to be—creamy, sweet, and cold. The best thing about it is that you can enjoy it any time you want without fear of setting back your healing. Ice cream for breakfast? Absolutely! Ice cream for dinner? Why not? It also makes the perfect snack. No matter when you enjoy your banana ice cream, your thyroid and the rest of your body will thank you for the healing benefits this indulgence brings.

3 large frozen bananas

2 cups defrosted wild blueberries, divided

2 tablespoons raw honey (optional)

Place 1 cup of thawed wild blueberries and their liquid into the food processor along with 2 tablespoons of raw honey if desired. Pulse 5 times until just combined. Many of the berries should still be whole. Set this sauce aside.

Roughly chop the bananas and place them into a food processor along with the remaining cup of wild blueberries. Process until a smooth soft-serve ice cream forms. If desired, you can place the ice cream into the freezer to harden for 2 hours before scooping it out.

Serve the ice cream in individual bowls and top with the wild blueberry sauce. Enjoy!

TIP

- Make this into an ice cream sundae with your choice of healing toppings. Try sprinkling your dish with chopped dates or figs, fresh berries, sliced banana, shredded coconut, hemp seeds, or chopped walnuts.

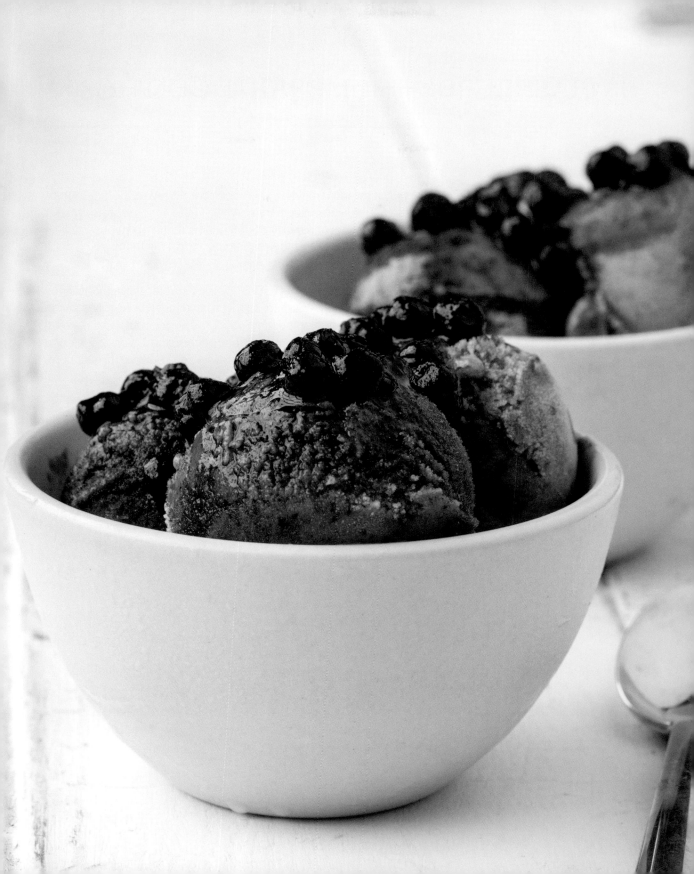

RASPBERRY THUMBPRINT COOKIES

Healing doesn't mean that you can't enjoy a sweet treat when you need one! These raspberry thumb-prints are delicious and have none of the harmful ingredients that can be found in some store-bought kinds. The bright pop of raspberry jam nestled in a rich, nutty dough makes these gorgeous cookies a true gift to yourself.

1 cup plus 2 tablespoons almond flour

½ teaspoon baking soda

½ teaspoon sea salt

½ cup tahini

½ cup coconut sugar or maple sugar

½ teaspoon alcohol-free vanilla extract

½ cup white sesame seeds

½ cup raspberry jam (see Tips, below)

Preheat the oven to 350°F. Whisk together the almond flour, baking soda, and sea salt in a mixing bowl and set aside. Process together the tahini, coconut sugar, and vanilla extract in a food processor until smoothly combined. Add the almond flour mixture to the food processor and pulse until well combined. If mixture is still crumbly, add water by the tablespoon as needed until smooth dough forms.

Form the dough into 1-inch balls and roll them in the sesame seeds before placing them onto a baking tray lined with parchment paper. Leave at least 2 inches between the cookies. Press a thumbprint into the center of each cookie and place the cookies into the oven. Bake the cookies for 8 to 10 minutes.

Remove the cookies from the oven and fill each one with 1 teaspoon of raspberry jam. Place the cookies on a wire rack to cool.

TIPS

- If using store-bought jam for filling, make sure to look for a clean one with no added harmful ingredients or preservatives.

- To make a homemade raspberry filling, mash fresh, ripe raspberries (or frozen raspberries that have been thawed) with raw honey or maple syrup until desired consistency is reached.

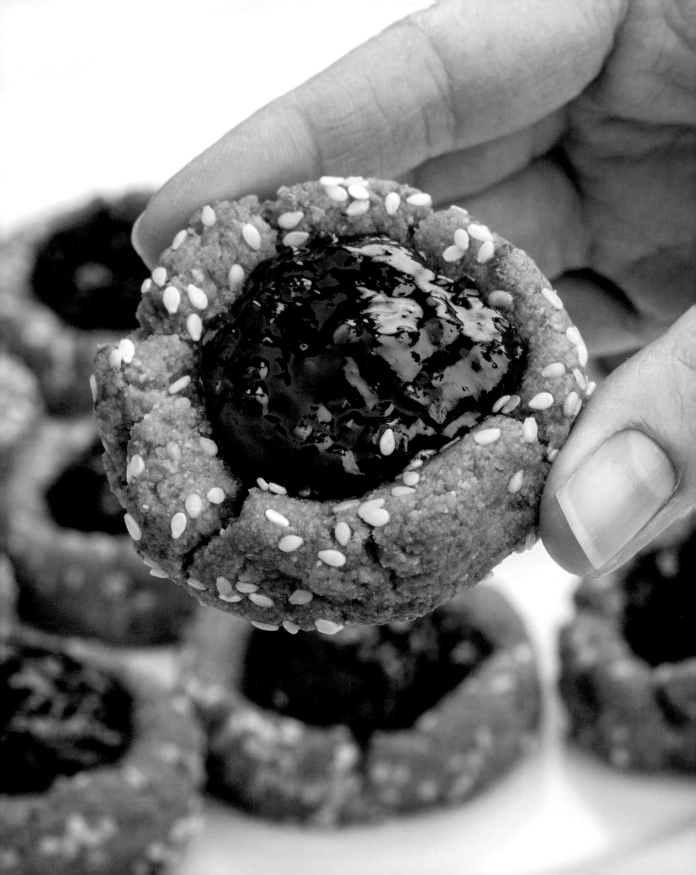

Thyroid Grab & Go Combos

Sometimes simple is all you need—or have time for. When you're running out the door or too busy to follow a recipe, you don't need to sacrifice nutrition or flavor for convenience. Instead, pull together these quick and easy food combinations specifically geared to support your healing process. Better yet, prep a few of these pairs ahead so that when time is of the essence, all you need to do is grab them and go.

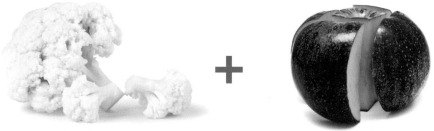

Cauliflower   *Apple*

- **Cauliflower florets + Apple slices:** this combination brings inflammation down in the thyroid while providing new memory to the thyroid's cells, teaching them to be independent after they may have grown sluggish from thyroid medication dependency.

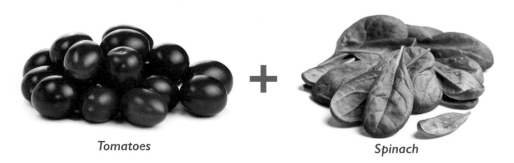

Tomatoes   *Spinach*

- **Tomatoes + Spinach:** together, these foods strengthen the liver at the same time that they flush the lymphatic system and build up the immune system to fend off a viral load that may target the thyroid.

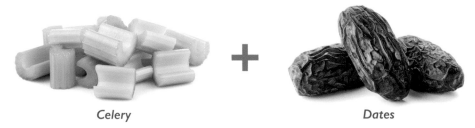

Celery   *Dates*

- **Celery + Dates:** combining critical mineral salts with high-quality, bioavailable glucose, this is a powerful adrenal restorative to provide backup superpower for the thyroid.

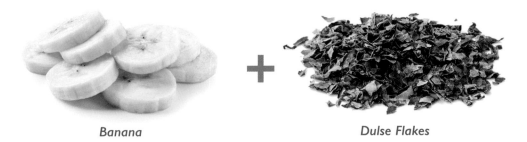

Banana   *Dulse Flakes*

- **Banana + Dulse flakes:** iodine, potassium, and sodium together in this snack strengthen the entire endocrine system and central nervous system against neurotoxins and their ill effects.

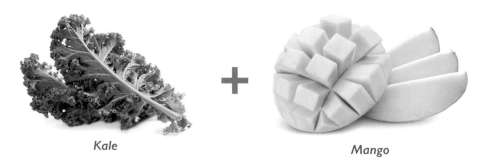

Kale   *Mango*

- **Kale + Mango:** this combination of alkaloids and carotenes allows them to easily enter the thyroid, helping to stop the growth of nodules and cysts there.

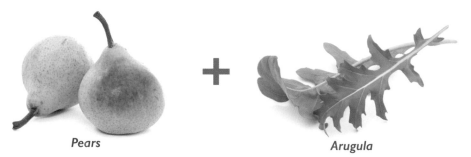

Pears   *Arugula*

- **Pear + Arugula:** wonderful for protecting the thyroid from atrophy and shrinkage. Together, these foods boost the thyroid's frequency abilities.

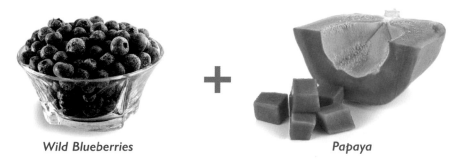

Wild Blueberries   *Papaya*

- **Wild blueberries + Papaya:** provide fighting power to stop, reduce, and prevent thyroid tumors (both cancerous and benign). Restore thyroid tissue after part of the gland has been surgically removed or killed off through radioactive iodine treatment.

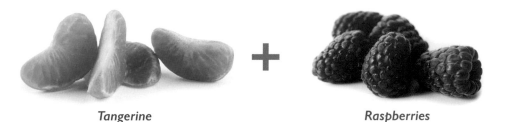

Tangerine   *Raspberries*

- **Tangerine + Raspberries:** as a team, these foods help prevent the calcium loss that can occur as the thyroid virus forces the body to use its calcium stores to wall off the virus in nodules and cysts, both in the thyroid itself and throughout the body. Help prevent osteoporosis.

CHAPTER 25

Thyroid Healing Techniques

If you came to this book with the belief that your thyroid had let you down or your body had somehow turned against you, it is vital to your healing process that you remind yourself each and every day now that your body is on your side.

Do whatever you need to do to internalize this message. Post a note on your bathroom mirror, write it in your journal each night, or make it a daily affirmation. You did nothing wrong. Your body did nothing wrong. Physically, emotionally, and spiritually, you are in sync in your intention to get better. When you really connect with this—when you understand that your thoughts and feelings were never holding you back, that your body was never attacking you—you activate healing on every level.

Throughout Part III, "Thyroid Resurrection," you've found knowledge and techniques to heal from the thyroid virus. In the following pages, you'll find techniques you can employ to activate healing specifically in your thyroid. These help the thyroid physically and also on a soul level—because your thyroid has its own soul, and when that soul is nurtured, your thyroid blossoms and thrives, just like the care and feeding of your greater soul is integral to your well-being.

LIGHT INFUSION TONICS

One powerful technique for relief and support when you're dealing with a thyroid condition is to infuse your drinking water with healing light. To do this, pour a glass of water and set it down in front of you. Raise a fist above your head, and visualize it filling with white light. Now release your hand, opening your fingers toward the glass, and say "Light" aloud as you picture the light streaming into the water. Repeat—making a fist again, gathering light, and then releasing it toward the glass as you say "Light"—for an ideal total of seven times. Angels around you will know what you're doing and assist you with the light making.

With each repetition, light infuses the water with more healing energy, changing its structure so that it becomes a divine, transformative tonic. For particular thyroid support, gargle the water before swallowing it. As you do so, envision the water's light flowing into your thyroid and killing off the EBV cells that are targeting the gland as it also repairs tissue damage.

Filling water with light is also a compassionate gesture if you're looking to support a loved one who's suffering with a thyroid condition. Follow the infusion process above, then offer it to your partner, friend, or family member.

Making light-filled water part of a thyroid-healing routine, whether you've infused it yourself or it's come from another, gives your thyroid a blanket of compassionate support. At the same time, the light stimulates the thyroid's personalized immune system, namely its special lymphocytes, and can act as a battery charger to the gland.

For some additional gentle thyroid hormone support, make your own homeopathic tonic by first mixing the water with the powdered amino acid supplement L-tyrosine and a bit of iodine. Add one quarter of the L-tyrosine bottle's recommended dosage to eight ounces of water, plus one tiny drop of high-quality, nascent iodine. Stir well, then follow the light infusion instructions above.

BUTTERFLY SUN SOAKING

You may have heard the shape of the thyroid gland compared to the shape of a butterfly. With a winglike lobe on either side, there is a similarity. Little does anyone know that it goes beyond looks.

In fact, the thyroid collects sunlight on those "wings" much like a butterfly does. (Plus butterflies fly on and produce radio-like frequencies, as the thyroid does.) When you soak up sunlight, especially when you get it on the front of your neck, even for just a few minutes, your thyroid collects it as though the gland were made of two solar panels. This sunlight helps power your thyroid, balances its production of hormones, keeps EBV from proliferating there, and stimulates and strengthens your thyroid's own immune system and your overall immune system, which in turn keeps the virus from doing damage to the thyroid.

All that and your thyroid also acts as your body's storage bin for the sun's rays. When you go days, weeks, or even months without getting enough sun, your immune system can pull from your thyroid's storage of that light and energy to defend your thyroid and the rest of your body against invaders like EBV.

To enhance your thyroid's process of collecting sunlight for healing, try this meditation:

As you sit in the sunlight, envision your thyroid as a butterfly resting on a rock. Feel each lobe—or "wing"—fan out in the warmth. Now see and feel the sun's rays absorbing into each wing, sending their healing energy deep into your cells.

As you do all this, breathe deeply and evenly. Feel yourself breathing light into your throat at the same time as air. As we talked about, getting enough oxygen is an important part of fighting off the thyroid virus. This deep breathing helps oxygenate your blood, which helps protect you from EBV.

If you're missing all or part of your thyroid, know that a butterfly can still fly with a torn wing; it runs on the butterfly's all-one energy provided by the earth's frequency. As we looked at earlier, when your thyroid is compromised or gone, your body still operates as if your thyroid were intact, so this technique still works.

It's an exercise that works when your thyroid is in perfect health, too, so long after you've said good-bye to EBV and any health concerns and brought your thyroid back to life, you can continue to return to this meditation as an act of thankfulness. Taking the time to honor your thyroid for all it has done for you, and to support it in supporting you, you'll also get a chance to reflect back on how far you've come.

TWO THYROIDS ARE BETTER THAN ONE

The thyroid's radio-like frequencies that we looked at in Chapter 4, "Your Thyroid's True Purpose," don't stop at communicating with the rest of the body. These frequencies also reach out to others' thyroids, which means that a healthy thyroid has the ability to support an ailing one simply by proximity.

Here's how it works: If someone with an ailing thyroid damaged by the thyroid virus stands next to someone with a better-functioning thyroid, the two thyroids will communicate with each other through their radio-like frequencies, with the ailing thyroid sending out a request for help. When the healthier thyroid detects this signal, it will first send a preliminary message to prime the compromised thyroid to receive aid. Once the thyroid in need has prepared itself, the helper thyroid will send a frequency that improves the ability of the other thyroid's personalized immune system (the lymphocytes in that area) to protect the gland and also assists the thyroid in receiving the lymphocytes' help, at the same time strengthening the thyroid itself. Even if you're missing your thyroid, it can receive help in this way—as we looked at in Chapter 20, "Life without a Thyroid," your thyroid still has a presence no matter what.

The frequencies that the thyroid emits are extremely powerful; they're similar to the messages that whales and dolphins use to communicate in the ocean. The thyroid's frequencies are so strong that if one person is developing thyroid cancer, another person's thyroid can send it messages to slow down and try to stop that cancer's development.

It takes close contact for two thyroids to communicate—the two people must be at most an arm's length apart. A hug is a great way for a thyroid to get or give help, though not the only way. As long as another person is within arm's reach, your thyroids' frequencies can get to each other. This thyroid-to-thyroid support will happen even if you don't love or even like one another. You could be sitting next to your boss in a meeting, a boss who's insulted you more times than you can count, and if her thyroid is in need and yours is doing better, yours will help hers—or vice versa.

You've probably experienced this thyroid communication phenomenon without knowing what it was. It's how unexplained feelings can come over you when you're in the presence of another person. It may be someone whose personality puts you off, and yet standing side-by-side in the break room at work, a warm, comfortable, at-ease feeling will wash over you, leading you to want to be around him. People don't realize in this situation that the feelings come either because your thyroid is offering help or receiving it.

Now imagine what this thyroid-to-thyroid communication can do for you when you know it's happening. The knowledge alone that you have this tool in your toolkit can strengthen and support your thyroid. The awareness that your thyroid is not on its own, that it can receive assistance from those around you, is an extraordinary technique to take the loneliness and despair out of illness. Even if you don't have the most supportive people in your life, their thyroids can help yours heal. Our thyroids are compassionate. They offer help unconditionally. Knowing that there's a part of us that operates with this unconditional compassion elevates our understanding of ourselves and each other, giving us hope and true appreciation for our internal workings.

And if you're the friend, family member, or caretaker of someone with thyroid illness, this gives you a way to know you are helping. It's so easy to feel powerless when we watch a loved one suffer. When you know that simply being close to someone with a compromised thyroid physically supports that person, you can have some peace.

You don't need to have a perfectly healthy or even intact thyroid yourself in order for it to offer help to another thyroid. In fact, you could be suffering with mild hypothyroidism yourself, and your thyroid will be able to send out healing frequencies to a thyroid that's in, for example, an advanced stage of Hashimoto's thyroiditis. All it takes is for one thyroid to be slightly healthier than the other. The only time that one thyroid can't support another is when their challenges are exactly equal, and that's very rare. Most of the time, even similarly compromised thyroids have subtle differences. This means that no matter how much you are suffering, you are probably still in a position to support someone who's worse off simply by being in their presence, giving you a way to help others when you're tired of being the one who needs help. The effects of one thyroid aiding another can last for days or even weeks.

All of this happens without draining the healthier thyroid. These messages don't take away from its own strength; the healthier thyroid doesn't take on the problems of the one in need. And as we looked at in Chapter 3, "How the Thyroid Virus Works," by the time EBV has caused damage to the thyroid, it's not contagious anymore, so being close to someone with a struggling thyroid won't hurt a person who's not dealing with the thyroid virus.

Medical research and science will not discover inter-thyroid communication (what I call *ITC*) for another hundred years or more, since they don't yet have basic awareness of the thyroid's radio-like frequencies within the body, let alone outside of it. For science to grasp this process, they'll need tests to detect and monitor the frequencies—tests that don't yet exist.

For now, have faith. In this moment, with all your new expertise, you've already begun to heal. You are the closest you've ever been to feeling better. That day when you can't remember what it feels like to be unwell is out there. Keep a light heart. Show yourself some compassion. And remember: you *can* heal.

CHAPTER 26

Finally Healed—
One Woman's Story

Sally Arnold knew she wanted to help people with their health since she was a small girl, so when she became a registered nurse as a young woman, it wasn't just a career, it was a calling. As she gained experience in the field, she never had a reason to doubt her training or colleagues. She worked with compassionate, intelligent people who made the lives of their patients better.

Sally had also had a few health challenges along the way, beginning with a hysterectomy and a prescription for hormone replacement therapy in her 20s. For the next 20-plus years, "autoimmune-ish" symptoms stayed with her. These included insomnia, severe exhaustion, a foggy brain (she always felt like it was three o'clock in the morning), weight gain (despite regular exercise and calorie restriction), chronic grumpiness, cold hands and feet, small growths on her skin, arthritis-like achiness in her joints, a chronic stuffy nose, lower libido, a feeling of slowness, chronic constipation that translated to bowel movements only twice a week, toenail fungus that turned her big toenail gray-black, forgetfulness, a pervasive gray-cloud feeling, irrational anxiety, and a racing heart that could go up to 120 beats per minute out of nowhere, sometimes prompting panic attacks that woke her in the middle of the night. She'd always had a buoyant, happy nature, so she imagined that the challenge of this mystery condition could have resulted in a deep depression for someone else.

Plus, Sally dealt with hair loss to the point of finding shiny bald spots on her scalp that felt like pencil erasers. At the hairdresser, she'd get tutorials on how to comb over and fluff up her hair to conceal the bare areas. Her eyebrows were falling out, too. She worried that she might eventually end up bald. Twice—only six weeks apart—she experienced labyrinthitis, inner ear inflammation that caused dizziness so strong that she had to visit the hospital and be wheeled into the ER while vomiting from the spinning. She also had a rash that had worked its way up to covering three-quarters of her back that no one knew how to address; she worried it would keep advancing. Everything felt big, and she felt raw and vulnerable.

For two decades, Sally didn't feel like herself. She exercised five times a week and watched what she ate, so she couldn't figure out why she didn't feel better. It didn't make sense. "As a nurse," she says, "I felt like I had failed my own health. I felt lonely inside my body."

Still, she didn't have a reason to believe that medical answers were missing. "How do you know what you don't know?" she says now. One doctor listened to her symptoms, described her in her chart as "obese, middle-aged, and female," and declared that she had Hashimoto's. Sally felt judged and unheard. She went along with his prescription for synthetic thyroid hormones, hoping that it would help her feel better. On the medication, though, her TSH test only came back at 0.24. She didn't experience any improvements—and in fact ended up with seven nodules on her thyroid.

Next, she went the holistic route. Going by a symptoms checklist rather than lab tests, this new doctor confirmed that her issues must be thyroid-related and switched her to porcine-derived thyroid medication.

Sally still didn't feel better. She visited another doctor, and he put her back on the synthetic thyroid hormones. Before long, though, she was back on the porcine thyroid hormones. She did this medication dance for years, scared of what would happen if she went off them, and all the while, her symptoms got worse, her hair kept falling out, and the size of her body grew. At various points, she had been told she had hyperthyroidism, hypothyroidism, and Hashimoto's. Nobody had the answers. The only thing Sally knew was that the doctors didn't know.

By the time she was 52, Sally was "sick and tired of feeling sick and tired." She'd tried the traditional medical approach, nothing worked, and she realized the medical field couldn't answer her questions about why she felt so poorly. That's when she contacted me. Despite feeling that talking to me was "pretty out there" and a big leap of faith considering her background as a clinical nurse, she was desperate for answers, and she was curious if I could tell her what was wrong.

Before our phone call, Sally wrote down a list of her questions for me. She was skeptical enough that she didn't want to offer any information, so instead, she let me do all the talking. Through listening to Spirit and doing my scan of her body, I found that EBV was at the root of her problems. It explained everything, from the achiness to the anxiety to the thyroid diagnoses to the inner ear inflammation to the rash to the irritability to the insomnia and beyond.

As I told her about her health, Sally says that I went down her private handwritten checklist item by item, in order, as if I had been reading it. At the end of my scan, I mentioned a small calcification in her left breast that she'd known about for over 15 years. It had been observed by mammogram, hadn't caused any problems, and no one other than her doctors and family knew about it. When I brought it up, she knew that she could trust the information I was offering.

In order to heal her EBV, I suggested that for a little while, Sally try cutting out the problematic foods that I list in Chapter 21, "Common Misconceptions and What to Avoid." In their place, I suggested that she load up on fruits and vegetables, with a focus on wild blueberries, kale, and cilantro. I also pointed her toward antiviral supplements such as L-lysine and, because I could tell she could tolerate it, small amounts of iodine.

As she began to feel better, Sally made the decision that she wanted to go off of the five different medications she was taking, including her thyroid prescription. Over the next year, she decided to lower her dosages incrementally, because she wanted to do it right. A few months after being medication-free, she went in for thyroid testing. Her TSH level was now 1.52, totally within the normal range, and her other lab values were normal, too, other than high cholesterol, which she'd had even when she was young and athletic. Taming EBV had brought her thyroid back to health.

Now, over two years since that first phone call, Sally says that her quality of life is "so much more harmonious." In the beginning, she wasn't sure how she would adapt to the change in diet, though it's now easy, normal, and no big deal. Her husband, who's been incredibly supportive all along, nonetheless used to laugh at the color of her morning detox smoothies; he now drinks one every day. She's thrilled to be able to eat fruit again after being scared of it for years, and she likes to approach meals with the question, "What can I eat today that's bright and colorful?" instead of "How will I get my servings of fruits and vegetables?"

Though most of her improvements were incremental, one was immediate: the relief of her constipation. Every morning since our phone call, she's had a bowel movement—which she says in itself was transformative after the discomfort that used to plague her. Symptoms like her toenail fungus were slower moving, though they did leave her eventually. Her thyroid nodules disappeared, and she hasn't had a panic attack in over two years.

Before lowering her EBV viral load, Sally's lower back had gone out on a regular basis, to the point where sometimes she couldn't even walk. Her husband, a chiropractor, had always said it didn't feel musculoskeletal, though they didn't know to relate it to her other symptoms. Now she can trace those back problems to viral flare-ups; her back hasn't gone out since

she started the protocol. The only change that hasn't come yet is losing some extra weight. To shed those unwanted pounds and enter her next phase of healing, Sally has just started juicing so she can alkalize and flush her system. (The bright side is that Sally's weight at least stabilized once she started fighting off EBV. If she hadn't gotten her EBV under control, she would have been become much heavier over the past two years.)

Some of Sally's greatest relief comes from the shift in her mental state. "It's really hard to be your best self when you're exhausted," she says, and now that the fatigue has lifted and she's able to sleep again, her short fuse is gone. She's back to being responsive rather than reactive and has returned to her default state of going to bed happy and waking up happy. She has the energy and enthusiasm to balance her family with caring for her property, running two cafés, and traveling often as she pursues the work of her heart, using her background in nursing to teach a neuroscience-based secular mindfulness curriculum.

A sense of well-being and peace has replaced Sally's anxiety and gray-cloud feeling. She feels so good, in fact, that she can easily forget how miserable and disconnected she used to feel, and how that was her normal. This past summer, she even went backpacking into the Emigrant Wilderness in California with a 45-pound pack for five days. Sally hadn't backpacked since she was 18. She feels like she got her life back. Her transformation makes her believe in the power of hope, intuition, baby steps, and following your internal compass. "Change will happen," she says. "Our bodies have the wisdom and know the way."

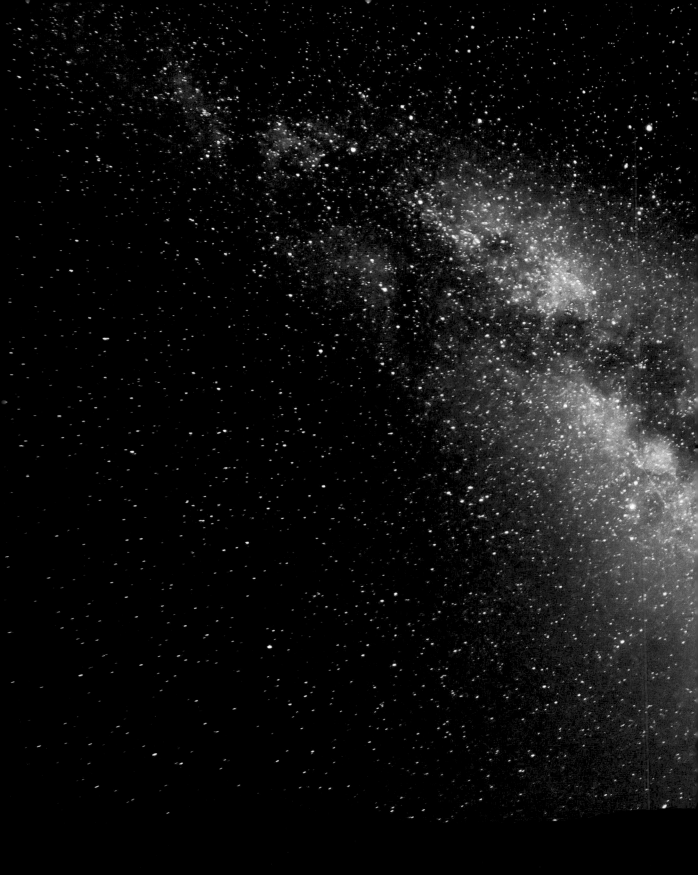

PART IV

SECRETS OF SLEEP

CHAPTER 27

Insomnia and Your Thyroid

If you struggle to get restful sleep, your thyroid is not the cause. You've probably heard the exact opposite, because the trends say that thyroid issues explain so much of insomnia. Truth is, they don't. If you find yourself tossing and turning at night, your thyroid is not to blame.

Sleep itself is still such a mystery to medical communities, so the reasons why sleep goes wrong for so many people are even more enigmatic to them. That's why certain theories crop up, like the idea that a compromised thyroid—another mysterious aspect of health—creates sleep disruptions. Blaming the thyroid like this is like arriving at the scene of a house fire and pointing to the chimney as the cause without doing any forensics. With the proper approach, investigators would find that there wasn't even a fire in the fireplace, and the boiler wasn't running—the chimney couldn't have been the cause. And yet because it's right there, it's considered the problem.

The thyroid-as-problem fad is not based on proof or understanding. It's mythical. Though as I've said before, myths can become law when they're repeated often enough. Not a single strand of truth could tie sleep and thyroid together. It just so happens that many people have both a sleep issue and a thyroid issue at the same time, so medical theorists have mistaken correlation for causation. In many cases, both thyroid problems and disrupted sleep are caused by the Epstein-Barr virus—which is the true reason they so often happen in tandem.

That's right; EBV is yet again a culprit in a common health complaint. It's not the only culprit, though. Many different factors can cause trouble with sleep, and you can have several going on at once. For example, EBV's neurotoxins may be diminishing the neurotransmitters you need to send the proper sleep signals; and at the same time, your liver may be clogged, which sends it into a subtle spasm in the early morning hours that wakes you up once you've finally fallen asleep. On top of which, maybe a lot of MSG has snuck its way into your meals over the years, and the MSG buildup in your brain is burning out the neurons you need to keep your mind at peace at bedtime.

Or maybe you're in the situation where EBV's neurotoxins are giving you aches and pains that make it difficult to sleep, plus your adrenals are too maxed out to produce enough of the specialized adrenaline blend you need to power sleep signals, plus some toxic heavy metals that have gotten into your system over the years are blocking proper sleep-related neurological activity in your brain.

More on these and other causes soon. Know this: In none of these cases is the thyroid itself the problem. Sleep is not governed by your thyroid hormones. Your thyroid is also not burning out your brain or clogging your liver or making you achy or antagonizing your adrenals or filling your system with toxins. It's innocent. Those who say otherwise are misled. The trend that says your thyroid explains sleep is one where two medical mysteries are combined as though two unknowns make a known. It's a situation where well-meaning practitioners adopt a theory as a belief system and put the idea out there, and the theory can quickly take on a life of its own.

Here's the thing: Sleep is critical for ridding yourself of EBV and healing your thyroid. As long as you go by the misguided theories, you'll be cut off from getting to the bottom of your sleep issue, and without understanding what's going wrong with your sleep, it's very difficult to make the problem go away.

Even if you wouldn't list insomnia or sleep disturbance as one of your chronic issues, learning how to harness sleep so it can be the most healing it can be is a critical part of your recovery. So far in this book, you've discovered the virus that's behind the vast majority of thyroid disorders, you've gained knowledge about the health mistakes and misconceptions to avoid, you've read all about foods and supplements that kill the virus and repair the thyroid, and you've picked up some techniques to take your healing even further. Now we arrive at the cornerstone: sleep.

Without the proper sleep, you can't properly heal. When you do get proper sleep, and when you know how to put your mind at ease when you're lying there awake, you possess one of the most powerful weapons for fighting EBV and resurrecting your thyroid.

That's because sleep is essential to immune function—your overall immune system and your thyroid's and liver's individual immune systems. It's the ultimate restorative, useful for (1) building up the thyroid's strength so it can keep the body in homeostasis as well as fend off and cleanse virus cells there, (2) bolstering the liver as it cleanses itself of EBV and its waste matter, and (3) allowing neurotransmitter chemicals to restore themselves after being burnt out by viral neurotoxins.

Sleep is an amazing preventative, too. For example, if you get the right sleep when EBV is still in Stage Two (plus you get the nutritional support we looked at in Part III, "Thyroid Resurrection," and remove those foods that feed the virus), your liver can get the support it needs to fight off the viral infection so that it doesn't advance to the thyroid.

If you struggle with sleep, this may all sound stressful. You may be thinking, *Enough already, I get it. Of course I would get sleep if I could*. Since the irony is that getting sleep helps heal the issues that cause problems with sleep in the first place, you may be worried that because sleep doesn't come easily for you, you're cut off from this precious resource. It can feel like a vicious cycle.

Set your worries aside. First of all, when you figure out what's behind your sleep issue in the first place, insomnia no longer has the power to loom over you as this unknowable adversary. When you can identify what's keeping you from the sleep you need, you gain the upper hand, and sleep immediately becomes less elusive. Secondly, there are secrets of sleep you can learn to employ to your advantage, so that its healing benefits don't remain out of reach.

When you see into sleep's mysteries, the cycle transforms from vicious to virtuous. The more quality sleep you get, the more you can eliminate the issues that make sleep troublesome in the first place. Around and around it goes as you heal, until sleep becomes your go-to source of respite—one that takes care of you and renews you so you can meet another day with the vitality you need to pursue your purpose and make the world a better place.

CHAPTER 28

Your Sleep Wellspring

We all want restful sleep. We all *deserve* restful sleep. From the moment you left the womb and took your first breath, sleep was owed to you. With every waking breath you've taken since, you've earned more sleep.

When I first came into my gift, I struggled to get much sleep. As a child and teenager, I was constantly up in the night worrying about the widespread suffering Spirit revealed to me. I was still getting used to seeing people's health problems everywhere I went. When my head hit the pillow come nightfall, I couldn't get it out of my mind. I didn't really feel like I deserved to rest when people were out there in pain.

Surviving on barely any sleep was its own version of hell. If you've struggled with insomnia, then you know what I'm talking about. To get me through that time, Spirit taught me about the laws of sleep and about secrets to making the most of what sleep I could get. It was critical information that helped me adapt to the challenges of my gift, and as I've shared it with others, it has provided them with major relief. This is information that you need, too.

There are so many negative messages about sleep out there. We hear, "You can sleep when you're dead," and, "No one ever accomplished anything by sleeping in." From the other side of the argument, we hear that we're not living up to our potential if we don't get at least eight hours of sleep a night. The competing ideas leave us spinning, not really sure if we should sleep less or more, and filled with guilt both if we oversleep *and* if we don't get our eight hours. We lose trust that the sleep we get is the "correct" sleep.

Sleep is not merely a physical function. It is a divine, metaphysical right. You should not feel guilty for getting as much sleep as you need, even if that means making sacrifices so you have the time. It's vital to the healing and adaptation of our bodies and souls. Which isn't to say that you should feel inadequate if you have trouble sleeping. It's not your fault. You're not just a "bad sleeper" and stuck that way for life. If you struggle with insomnia or the sleep you get doesn't feel restorative, read on. I share secrets in this chapter about how you claim your right and make the most of what rest time you do get.

Medical communities do not yet have a grip on how sleep works. It's one of the great cosmic mysteries, along with what happens to food when it enters the stomach. Unlike a broken leg or a diseased kidney, it's intangible, out of reach. Sometimes we get distracted from how science does not yet have all the answers. We hear terms like *REM* and *circadian rhythms*, read about sleep studies and brain waves, and it makes us think that current knowledge is a bit more advanced than it is.

Sleep is still a medical guessing game. It is still widely misunderstood, which means that sleep issues aren't grasped yet, either. Today's sleep treatments waver between drinking a glass of warm milk before bed and taking dangerous sleeping drugs to knock yourself out. Research is as much as 500 years away from understanding scientifically how sleep works. It's like those early days of the computer: In 1959, when a computer was the size of a house and could perform only a few core functions, we thought we were on top of the world. Now we carry computers in our pockets that run our lives. Looking back, we realize how far we still had to go back then, when we thought we were advanced.

It's important to have the full scope on sleep, because there are all sorts of reasons that people have difficulty sleeping, and they are very real. There's worry and sadness. There's overstimulation from so much screen time, a concept that's gaining popularity in news articles on health. Sleep apnea is a condition that's getting more attention lately, too, though what causes some forms of it still leaves people at a loss. Anxiety interferes with sleep, though the answers aren't out there about why it exists in the first place or how to curb it. Then there are underlying conditions that no one thinks about as causing sleep interruptions—we're talking a sluggish liver, a sensitive intestinal lining, and adrenal fatigue. And not to be underestimated are heightened levels of toxic heavy metals and MSG that interrupt brain and nerve signals. Finally, of course, we have viral issues like EBV activity. As I mentioned, this is one of the most frequent explanations behind troubled sleep. We'll look at all of this and more in the pages to come, including how to deal with a sleepless night and what bad dreams really mean.

If we're going to keep up with this time that Spirit calls the Quickening—when the pace of life is faster than ever before in history—it's critical that we connect with the secrets of sleep. After all, sleep is a time of sacred communion with the divine to help us heal and adapt to this crazy world. Before you can address an issue with sleep, you need to understand on a soul level how much you've earned it. So first, let's look at the basic laws of sleep. Forget about sleep hell. We're going to make sleep heavenly.

LAWS OF SLEEP

The foundation of a good night's sleep is to own the fact that it is your right. Somehow, we lose sight of this. We think that sleep is only for the lucky, the privileged, the deserving. However, sleep knows no bounds. Simply by existing as a human being, you have earned sleep. The laws of sleep cannot be amended. The right to sleep cannot be infringed upon or granted to only a certain class. By studying the laws below, you can start to take advantage of your birthright now. And over time, the knowledge can sink in on a core level: sleep is for you.

Your Sleep Wellspring

We often hear the term *sleep debt*. Just a mention of the term can put us in a funk; it's depressing to feel like we get more and more behind every time we lose a few hours of shuteye. For anyone who has trouble sleeping or finding the time to sleep, the concept is yet one more stressor.

Truth is, we each have a *sleep wellspring*. It is divine law that with every waking breath you take, you're delivered two seconds of sleep to use at any time you wish. Picture this sleep supply as flowing into a well that you have access to anytime you want for the rest of your life. It's not money, so you can never lose what builds up. The Holy Source and the Earthly Mother watch over this never-failing wellspring that God created for you when your life was created—it is part of your life force. Drought will never come to it. It can never be poisoned. All that can happen is that you dip into it when you want to sleep, and because you continue to earn more sleep every time you take a breath during your waking hours, you continuously replenish your supply. Whenever you miss sleep, it stays there in the well, waiting for the day when you can use it, even if that's ten years later.

This universal law can never be taken from you. No one has the right to rob you of your sleep. When you are having a conflict with a friend, family member, or co-worker that keeps you lying awake at night, that sleep you might have gotten isn't gone forever—no one stole it. Worry itself cannot take sleep from you. Not even the Epstein-Barr virus has the power to steal your sleep as it disrupts your neurotransmitters and keeps you from tapping into your sleep wellspring for a night. Any missed sleep is yours alone to reclaim another time. This isn't town water that's contaminated or filled with chlorine and fluoride, or that can be shut off if the water main breaks or you don't pay your bill. While conflicts, illness, and stress may make it difficult to access your sleep wellspring on a given night, sleep will still flow into your well, building up this clean, pure, natural, and spiritual resource for you to use later.

It's time for us to stop thinking of ourselves as sleep poor. All-nighters when you were in college, sleepless months when your children were infants, tossing and turning as you struggled with illness—you haven't been digging yourself deeper and deeper, beyond help, with every missed opportunity for a full night's sleep. You can always go back and get access to the sleep you couldn't use at an earlier time. We are rich in sleep.

Your Sleep Allowance

Knowing that you have this wellspring is one thing. Giving yourself permission to use it is another. Sometimes people don't allow themselves to sleep. It happens for a lot of reasons: a lack of trust that you deserve it; a lack of trust that you *can* sleep; a belief that you're not working hard enough to warrant it; or a fear of nightmares, or not being alert to your surroundings, or missing out on something going on in the waking world. People often feel that sleep is a luxury, and that you have to earn it. There are also creative types whose passion keeps them alert when they try to lie down, and so for fear of losing an idea, they keep the fires in their minds burning.

If you have trouble letting yourself sleep, then it's important to grant yourself a sleep allowance. It is law that you deserve this. This isn't like a child's allowance, where the kid is supposed to learn responsibility from imposed limits. It's more like if you invented some crazy-popular gadget that was selling like hotcakes, making you more money every day, and so to make yourself feel comfortable that you weren't going to squander all your earnings, you allowed yourself a daily draw. Knowing that you had this set amount of your earnings to use every day, you could relax with the knowledge that your fortune wasn't going to disappear.

It is okay to draw from your sleep wellspring—you truly *deserve* to use it. So every evening when you're getting ready for bed, do a little active meditation where you pour yourself a glass of water for the night and imagine that you're tapping into your sleep well at the same time. Like water from a faucet, sleep is meant to flow. And just as you can't survive if you cut yourself off from water, neither can you carry on if you don't give yourself permission to benefit from this resource. Sleep is yours to use, with no fear of running out. The wellspring will continue to replenish every day of your life.

CHAPTER 29

Identifying Sleep Issues

Sometimes there's no mystery about what's behind a night of troubled sleep. If, say, your teenager is out late at a party, then you know exactly why your mind's still whirring when you'd normally turn out the light. If you've recently gone through a breakup or had a disagreement with your partner, if you're worried about a big test or meeting the next morning, if you're grieving from a loss or an experience that broke your trust, or even if you're bursting with excitement for the day to come, you already know what's behind your insomnia.

Then there are those nights when none of the above is going on, or when it's in the background enough that you can shut it off when you click off the light. That puts you in the department of mystery sleep issues. Sometimes the most stressful part of this is the mystery, the not knowing what's behind the problem. A certain anxiety starts to creep in as the day dims, because you can't predict what the night ahead holds. Will this be one of those nights where you get through unscathed, lost in peaceful slumber until it's time to get up? Or will it be a night of torture where you fear with each passing hour you're awake that you'll be groggier and less alert for the day that follows? If it's not an anxiety disorder that's keeping you up, the unpredictability of an issue with sleep can give you one.

Sleep studies are a common technique used in the medical world to determine what's going on when someone's sleep is troubled. You visit a sleep lab, get hooked up to diodes, then try to drift off to sleep with technicians in the other room to monitor your body activity. Afterward, your doctor assesses the results to see if a sleep disorder is apparent.

Unfortunately, sleep studies rarely provide answers about what's really wrong and how to fix it. In the case of sleep apnea, for example, the condition in which breathing is interrupted or too shallow during sleep, a sleep study can be very helpful in diagnosing the apnea and determining its severity. A patient will then get a prescription for a continuous positive airway pressure (CPAP) machine with directions on which settings to use—and that's it. The CPAP may make some difference. It may even help greatly. The difference it makes in how the patient feels after a night of sleep may seem like, well, night and day.

What about the *cause* of the sleep apnea, though? What if the patient wants to alleviate the underlying condition that's giving her or him trouble breathing during sleep in the first place? Often, the best advice medical communities have to offer is to try to lose weight. (More on sleep apnea later.) So sleep studies have their limits.

If you want to address a sleep issue, the first step is to identify its characteristics. When it comes to troubled sleep, there isn't just one kind, so it can't all be explained and addressed in the same way. Here are some common issues people encounter with sleep:

- You can't fall asleep at first, then you finally nod off after several hours. When you wake up, you don't feel rested.

- You fall asleep easily, then wake in the wee hours, unable to fall back asleep before it's time to get up. Frustration at not being able to doze off again exacerbates your already racing mind, and when the sun starts to rise, it kicks up even more anxiety.

- As above, you fall asleep easily, then wake during the night, though in this case, you're able to fall back asleep eventually, in the early morning hours.

- You're in and out of a miserable sleep all through the night, never falling into a solid, restful sleep state. Frequent urgency to urinate can sometimes accompany this.

- You're up all night, and not because you want to be. You're not out partying, falling in love, or studying for an exam—you're in bed, suffering through the entire night with insomnia. When the morning comes, you're completely out of it, and you crash at various points during the day, though

napping may feel beyond reach. At night, you start the whole thing over again.

- All throughout the day, you're exhausted. You struggle through your tasks, and all you can think about is getting a chance to lie down and close your eyes. When the nighttime hits, suddenly you're "awake," and it's difficult to wind down enough to get to sleep on time.

- You're able to fall asleep and stay asleep for a full night, only you wake up feeling like you need another eight hours. This can go in two directions: (1) Your loved ones report that you snore loudly and/or that you stop breathing or breathe very shallowly during the night. They may even report that you woke yourself up snoring, though you immediately returned to sleep and didn't remember. (2) You've ruled out breathing problems, and the exhaustion persists. No matter how early you go to bed or how late you wake up, you don't feel refreshed after sleep.

- Just as you you're about to sink into sleep, an involuntary jerk of your arm or leg wakes you up again. This can happen several times in a row.

- You're tired and ready for sleep, except a background sensation keeps you awake. This can range from neurological (tinnitus, a buzzing feeling, restless legs syndrome) to skin problems to aches and pains to racing thoughts.

Once you've put a finger on what defines your sleep issue, you can move forward to determine which causes could be behind it.

CAUSES OF SLEEP ISSUES

Many factors, sometimes in combination with one another, can contribute to a person's inability to get a good night's rest. We hear a lot about how our devices keep us up with their unnatural light and brain-stimulating content. That's certainly one element to consider, and one that you've probably addressed if you struggle with sleep. You know to keep computers, phones, tablets, and alarm clocks away from your bed, to keep your bedroom dark and quiet, and to start winding down for bed with plenty of time beforehand.

What if you've tried all that, and your sleep issue remains a mystery? Not surprisingly, the Unforgiving Four of radiation, toxic heavy metals, viruses, and DDT, as well as some of their sidekicks and offshoots, play a role.

Viral Activity

Viral issues are one of the major causes of trouble with sleep. The Epstein-Barr virus, shingles, cytomegalovirus, HHV-6, and even some bacteria can poison our systems and keep us up at night. That's because viruses such as Epstein-Barr excrete neurotoxins, which are disruptive in three main ways: (1) They trigger hypersensitivity in the central nervous system, which governs sleep; (2) they create body aches and pains, which can prevent you from relaxing

enough to sleep; and (3) they can diminish neurotransmitter activity—and because your neurotransmitters allow for communication across brain cells, this can get in the way of the proper sleep messages getting through. In this way, viral neurotoxins can create the issues of not being able to fall asleep for hours, or waking in the middle of the night and not being able to fall back asleep.

Viral-caused insomnia is often mistaken for a thyroid issue, because, as I said earlier, it's common to experience insomnia and thyroid trouble side by side. It's not because an under- or overactive thyroid causes sleep issues, despite what you may hear from other sources. The reality is that a compromised thyroid and difficulty sleeping are both symptoms of EBV—that's the reason they coexist. Often, it's the thyroid virus in Stage Four causing the insomnia, which means a thyroid problem is already well underway, whether it's been detected at the doctor's office or not.

Toxic Heavy Metals

High on the list of sleep disturbers is having toxic heavy metals in the system. These heavy metals are especially problematic in the brain, where they don't just stay in one place; they oxidize, creating waves of toxic runoff, which spreads the metals and damages brain tissue in its path. Heavy metals can also short out electrical impulses and create problems with electrolytes and neurotransmitter chemicals, resulting in shutdown of the neurotransmitters that would otherwise send proper sleep messages throughout your brain. This dysfunction can cause a multitude of sleep issues, including erratic sleep, not getting deep sleep, and not being able to fall asleep in the first place.

Teenagers especially can be affected by toxic heavy metals interfering with sleep.

MSG Toxicity

A huge part of the country doesn't sleep because of MSG toxicity. This common ingredient goes straight to the brain, where it derails electrical activity with toxins and co-toxins that burn out brain tissue. And once MSG is in the brain, it stays there (unless you break it down and pull it out with detoxification techniques), creating long-term problems that can include trouble sleeping. That's because MSG is a neuron antagonist. It sticks to neurons and makes them electrically hypersensitive, so that when an electrical impulse moves through the neuron, it burns hotter, which causes an erratic, disproportionate reaction. It's as though the MSG makes the neuron into a sparkler. And like a sparkler, a neuron with this fuel-like coating of MSG eventually burns out.

MSG neuron antagonism can create rapid thoughts, a sense of itchiness, difficulty calming the mind, and the feeling of being obsessed about something you can't shake at bedtime. Many people who need to do a lot of meditation or calming techniques before settling down for the night, or who are constantly waking up throughout the night, have a higher amount of MSG saturating their brain tissue.

MSG is everywhere, so beware. As we looked at in my previous two books, one of the most deceptive places it hides is in the ingredient *natural flavors*, which can sneak into even the healthiest-looking packaged organic foods and supplements at the natural foods store. (For a fuller list of how MSG disguises itself in ingredients lists and restaurant food, see the chapter "What Not to Eat" in my first book.)

Liver Issues

Your liver works hard for you all day long. It fends off pathogens and toxins by purifying your blood and creates bile to break down excess fats in the diet. Just like you, the liver needs time to rest, and so when you go to bed at night, your liver goes to sleep, too. It shuts down operation for a while and goes into autopilot. By around three or four in the morning (it's different for everyone), your liver starts to wake up again. With that rejuvenating sleep it's just gotten, it once more begins to process poisons, bacteria, viruses, and debris (such as dead cells, including dead red blood cells), gathering them up like it's taking the trash out to the curb—so that when you wake up in the morning and get hydrated, you'll flush all of it out. This healing, cleansing process also prevents bilirubin accumulation.

If the liver is sluggish due to a diet too high in fat and processed foods, then as it tries to do its job in the wee hours of the morning, it goes into subtle spasm, squeezing and twisting around. Most of the time, it's not anything you can feel. However, the liver's little dance creates enough of a disturbance in the body that you can awaken. This accounts for those nights when you fall asleep normally, then suddenly you're up again in the early morning hours, and after a certain period of time, you're able to nod off again. This can also explain those miserable nights of sleep where you drift in and out the whole time.

Digestive Issues

Similarly, digestive issues can interfere with sleep. The nervous system is very sensitive and works in tandem with the digestive tract.

Your body's north-south (brain-gut) connectors known as the vagus and phrenic nerves mean that whatever's going on in your digestive tract is immediately signaled to your brain. So if you're someone with digestive pain, bloating, cramping, or a sensitive stomach, those symptoms can trigger off the nervous system and keep you alert when you're trying to sleep.

Digestive activity can also wake you up even if you don't feel any discomfort. A person often has no idea that, say, the ileum (the part of the small intestine that connects to the large intestine) is inflamed from excess adrenaline, and so whenever food passes through this stretch, it sets off nerves that connect to the brain. As you blink awake blearily into the dark, you won't be able to detect anything going on in your abdomen, and it will feel like you woke for no reason. Really, dinner has been digesting during sleep, and peristalsis has just caused food in the digestive tract to pass through a sensitive area.

Emotional Wounds

Oftentimes in our lives, we get let down. A best friend turns against you, a soul mate goes in another direction, your parents divorce, your body becomes sick with seemingly no explanation, those around you imply that you're to blame for your illness. With all of these experiences, we lose trust. And if a trust loss is big enough, or if too many trust breaks accumulate over time without being balanced out, we can experience emotional wounds. They're not merely emotional, though—there's also a physical component. As I revealed in the chapter "Posttraumatic Stress Disorder" in *Medical Medium*, traumas big and small can create neural burnout and scar brain tissue. The result is a large package put together with a big red bow of no sleep. So many experience this in their lifetime, and it's never any fun. For some, it can be devastating to their sense of who they are as a person and to the ones around them. As difficult as it can be, we can become empowered from these experiences along the way, recharge our souls, and rise out of the ashes of emotional wounds and PTSD.

Sleep Apnea

As I said earlier, sleep apnea is one sleep-related condition that medical research has started to piece together. In the past ten years, an increasing number of people have gotten sleep apnea diagnoses, and even TV shows now make jokes about middle-aged characters and their CPAP machines. Scientists have discovered that chronic snoring is not innocuous. It's often indicative of breathing problems that prevent someone from entering a truly restful sleep cycle, so doctors have started prescribing those CPAPs to force air through patients' airways while they sleep.

It's a great approach for someone with obstructive sleep apnea, which can result from a number of physical blockages. Some common causes of obstructive sleep apnea include excess mucus, as in postnasal drip; inflamed and expanded mucous membranes in the throat; inflammation of the bronchial tubes, tonsils, or adenoid; septum issues; chronic sinusitis; lymphatic obstruction; general swelling; edema; and excess weight that puts pressure on the throat and chest. As with all the other sleep issues we've looked at here, obstructive sleep apnea is not a life sentence—it's all about antiviral, anti-mucus, anti-inflammatory foods to give you relief.

There's also non-obstructive sleep apnea, which I call neurological sleep apnea. This is the form of the condition where a CPAP doesn't offer as much relief, because it's not just about the need to push air through; it's about the central nervous system and supporting nerves. Neurological sleep apnea overlaps with the sleep disorder that medical communities call central sleep apnea—which remains by and large a medical mystery. While research has identified central sleep apnea as distinct, it is still light years from understanding what's at the root.

Here's what's really going on when blockages aren't to blame for trouble breathing during sleep: for one, borderline seizure-like activity in the brain (caused by pollutants). These aren't actual seizures—rather, electrical power surges are occurring in the brain on a truly minute level. It's just enough to cause a pause in breathing. This type of neurological sleep apnea can occur as a result of MSG toxicity, high levels of a combination of toxic heavy metals such as mercury and aluminum, or exposure to pesticides such as DDT and/or herbicides. All of these factors are prone to creating chemical imbalances in the brain that cause these power surges. A common scenario is that someone develops sleep apnea after moving—and has no idea that it's due to the pesticides sprayed indoors by the former residents of her or his home. Viral activity can also cause neurological sleep apnea, because viral neurotoxins can inflame the vagus nerve, which runs through the chest and affects breathing.

Adrenal Fatigue

People who have never dealt with adrenal fatigue probably hear the word *fatigue* and think that for people who suffer with this condition, sleeping is the least of their worries. After all, doesn't fatigue just mean you're extra tired and could sleep at any time? Anyone who has dealt with persistent fatigue can tell you that this isn't the case. In fact, adrenal fatigue can set you up for *trouble* with sleeping. The condition is characterized by adrenal glands that swing between producing too much adrenaline and too little of it.

A common scenario is that the adrenal glands are underactive during the day, because they're holding back in case a crisis arises, and so you feel sluggish or a continual need to crash throughout the day. When the night comes and no emergency has occurred, the adrenals release the adrenaline they were holding on to, accounting for that "suddenly awake" feeling when the sun sets. It may also be that when your adrenals are overactive, they push out surges of corrosive excess adrenaline, which burns out and diminishes neurotransmitters, getting in the way of sleep.

Even underactive adrenals at night can make sleep problematic, because it means they may not be producing enough of the specific blend of hormone you need to fall asleep. (That's right—you need certain types of adrenaline for help with falling asleep, entering REM sleep, and dreaming.)

Anxiety

Were you one of those children who put off bedtime because you didn't want to be left alone in the dark? Or do you ever have trouble sleeping because something unpleasant is scheduled for the next day, and you don't want it to come too soon? We've all been there with sleep-related anxiety, even if only now and again. For some people, that anxiety is a regular occurrence, and it's usually not a mystery that worry and unease are behind their insomnia.

The question is, what's behind the unexplained sleep anxiety? In some cases, it's a fear of nightmares. In other cases, there's an element of PTSD or OCD involved: One of the other factors in this section has caused you enough trouble with sleep that your bed doesn't feel like a safe place, and you can't fully relax. For this type of situation, the underlying health issue is what needs to be addressed first, to eliminate any ongoing trauma or trigger.

In yet other cases, though, the anxiety is amorphous and unnameable and can't be traced to a specific triggering experience. This type of anxiety, similar to what we looked at in Chapter 5, "Your Symptoms and Conditions—Explained" has to do with the Unforgiving Four triggering physiological (often neurological) disturbances. In one type of anxiety, nerves become "allergic" to viral neurotoxins, which heightens nerve sensitivity and creates extreme feelings of anxiousness. In another scenario, toxic heavy metals oxidizing in the brain interrupt electrical impulses, causing them to ricochet, so that you experience panic, irrational thoughts, restlessness, or the sensation of not being able to think straight, because the messages in your brain aren't reaching their intended destinations.

Anxiety can also occur as a result of DDT in the brain. This pesticide that we think of as long gone is so tenacious that we're still dealing with it today, and it is a neuron antagonist that causes these nerve cells to self-destruct, which results in sudden feelings of anxiousness. Radiation, too, can contribute to sleep-disrupting anxiety, because radiation elevates histamine reactions and inflammation in the body—inflammation that's undetectable in classic inflammation blood tests such as C-reactive protein and antinuclear antibody tests. People with radiation-induced inflammation may feel hot or swollen, or their skin may slightly burn, all of which can result in an anxious, out-of-sorts state of mind that keeps sleep from coming easily.

And sometimes, anxiety kicks up because of something going on in the gut. As we looked at in "Digestive Issues" above, nerve connections mean that digestive sensitivity signals the brain. This is a common reason that someone can wake up worried for no apparent reason in the middle of the night. Depending on the level of intestinal irritation, they may be able to fall back asleep after it's passed, or they may be up for the duration once woken.

Additional Neurological Issues

For those who struggle to get even a wink of sleep all night, the cause is often serious neurotransmitter and neuron dysfunction, coupled with overactive or underactive adrenals. It can result in those undesired all-nighters, where even though you go to bed at a reasonable hour, you're still awake to see the sun rise. A severe lack of magnesium is often in play. And usually, this type of sleep distress has a foundation of PTSD. It's not the insomnia-induced PTSD I referenced a few pages ago—rather, it stems from a traumatic experience in some other area of life, whether in the distant or recent past, that has resulted in neurological issues. In this case, instead of running too hot, as in MSG toxicity, electrical impulses run too cold and become underactive. Without enough electricity moving through the neurons, the neurotransmitter chemicals, which are already depleted in such a circumstance, don't get enough "push" to send sleep messages to the brain cells.

And another neurological issue is repeated, involuntary jerking. This often means that the brain tissue is saturated with toxins such as toxic heavy metals, aspartame, MSG, DDT and other pesticides, herbicides, toxic nanomaterials, and/or other synthetic chemicals. Information is meant to travel through the brain gently and smoothly, on an ongoing basis. However, saturation means that the brain tissue is not quick to receive information from the neurotransmitters, and so the neurotransmitter chemicals get hung up and collect in small deposits until so much information builds up that they release that information in an unexpected spurt that jerks the body awake. (During the day, the same process happens to people who suffer from this condition, though they're not calm enough to sense it, because they're running on adrenaline. If they were to take a midday nap, though, they'd likely experience the same jerking.)

None of which is meant to worry you. All of the issues I've just listed can heal. The scary and disheartening part is not knowing what's going on, and feeling like it's out of your control. That's behind you. Now you have answers, and as I always say, that's the first step in healing. Let's explore how you can finally move forward.

CHAPTER 30

Healing Sleep Issues

What do we do about the issues from the previous chapter? How do we translate answers about what's behind our sleep deprivation into answers about how to let the sleep wellspring flow? Food is, of course, fundamental. Life-changing foods can change everything for you sleep-wise, which is why shortly, you'll get to a list of the best ones to incorporate into your life (along with which supplements they enhance). First, let's look at the particulars of healing from those sleep issues.

If you're dealing with viral infection, toxic heavy metals in the system, MSG toxicity, or any other toxic overload, then you want to make detoxification your first priority. Increasing the amount of fruits, vegetables, herbs, spices, and wild foods in your diet will automatically start your body on the path of detox. If your sleep problems are severe and you want to take your purification to the next level, then you'll find support in the 90-Day Thyroid Rehab. If EBV is the virus you're battling, you've already learned so much about how to tame the virus—which will translate to better sleep.

For specific conditions such as a sluggish liver, adrenal fatigue, and digestive issues, the best approach is to find the foods in Chapter 22 and in my second book that address those conditions. For a sluggish liver, for instance, lemon water first thing in the morning is a powerful technique to help the organ flush itself of buildup. When you do this on a regular basis, the liver has less work to do at night, which means a lower chance of going into spasm and waking you up. Also, the liver becomes sluggish in the first place due to factors such as an oversized viral load, excess fat in the diet, and heavy metal overload—all of which result in an inability to absorb and convert nutrients—so lowering dietary fat, flushing the liver with morning lemon water, and pampering your liver with fruits, vegetables, herbs, spices, and wild foods will help perk it up again.

For adrenal fatigue, grazing (that is, eating every one and a half to two hours) is key. You don't want to limit yourself to just two or three meals a day, because your adrenal glands end up having to dump adrenaline into your system when your blood sugar drops. When they get strained like that, your adrenals are much more likely to be over- or underactive come nighttime. You'll also want to limit adrenalized foods in your diet (see the chapter "Fertility and Our Future" in my second book) for the best chance of keeping the glands on an even keel so you can get some peace at night. If you want more help with adrenal fatigue, I devoted an entire chapter to the condition in *Medical Medium*.

And for digestive issues, in addition to paging through the options in *Medical Medium Life-Changing Foods*, you want to make elevated biotics your priority. These microscopic, life-giving organisms cover the above-ground surfaces (leaves and skins) of raw, unwashed (or lightly rinsed) organic produce. The elevated biotics' probiotic film can make a world of difference when it comes to digestion, filling in for some of the soil depletion we looked at in "Concerns about Zinc" in Chapter 21. Unlike factory-produced probiotics and soil-borne organisms, elevated biotics are able to survive your digestive process and make it to your ileum, the final section of your small intestinal tract that creates the vitamin B_{12} critical to your body's functioning. This doesn't mean that you have to start eating entirely raw foods. All it takes is supplementing your existing diet with fresh, raw, organic produce. Be selective and use your instincts about what produce you eat without washing. If you have a wax-covered, conventionally grown apple from the grocery store, you definitely want to scrub it before eating. It's not a good source of elevated biotics anyway, because the wax and pesticides used in the growing process have already interfered with the natural film of beneficial microorganisms. If, on the other hand, you have a piece of chemical-free, contaminant-free produce you'd like to eat that has visible dirt on it, a light rinse with plain water is usually fine—the elevated biotic film should stay intact (after all, the microorganisms survive rainfall). Sprouts that you grow on your kitchen countertop are an easy, elevated-biotic-rich source that you can sprinkle on your salads and wraps, or throw into smoothies. Otherwise, turn to your own organic garden or a local organic farmer you trust. The

"Gut Health" chapter in *Medical Medium* offers more resources for digestive healing.

If you're dealing with obstructive sleep apnea, all of the foods on the next pages help to reduce mucus, inflammation, and histamine production. And for neurological sleep apnea, these foods also support neurotransmitters with their higher levels of easily absorbable and assimilable amino acids.

In the case of anxiety, the best first step you can take is to add some true comfort foods to your life. Herbal tea with raw honey, a baked sweet potato with avocado—life-changing foods along these lines can offer you some emotional ease as you work through what's causing your anxiety. If nightmares are behind a sleep aversion, turn to the next chapter for an explanation of why bad dreams are actually a good sign.

If the source of your anxiety is harder to pin down, know that it's not your fault. Too many people with anxiety are made to feel like they're nuisances, and that they should just buck up and look on the bright side of life. The truth is, anxiety is very real, and underlying causes range from viral infection to trauma to electrolyte deficiency. In addition to the foods in this list, focus on those foods listed as helpful for alleviating anxiety in my second book.

For neurological sleep issues in general, the foods here apply for the same reasons I've just listed—they cleanse toxins, address nutrient deficiencies, and calm the brain and body. They also provide antioxidants and the critical glucose and mineral salts needed to produce neurotransmitter chemicals effectively and feed your brain in the best possible way—so you can finally get some sleep.

FOODS FOR SLEEP

The following foods address all of the conditions I've mentioned in this chapter, plus they enhance the effects of sleep-promoting supplements. In addition to the list below, focus on making berries, dates, lemons, limes, potatoes, radishes, turmeric, ginger, coconut water, sprouts, lemon balm, cat's claw, raw honey, artichokes, avocados, and grapes a part of your life.

You'll notice that many of these foods overlap with the ones in Chapter 22. That's the magic of these life-changing foods—they are multifaceted and adjust to your various individual needs at any given time. This also means that you don't need to worry that you can't eat the foods in this list during the day for fear they'll make you sleepy. Whatever time of day you eat these foods, they'll gear themselves to what's right for you in the moment.

- **Mangoes:** Very high in bioavailable magnesium. Eat one before bed to ease the transition to sleep. When you take supplemental **L-glutamine**, mangoes heighten its absorption, which reduces MSG toxicity by disarming it.

- **Bananas:** High in tryptophan and fructose to soothe neurotransmitters. When combined with **5-HTP**, bananas activate the supplement, which allows for higher bioavailability and quicker absorption of it.

- **Cherries:** A great source of melatonin, a nutrient-based hormone that helps your neurotransmitters and glial cells.

When you eat cherries at the same time you take supplemental **melatonin**, the cherries heighten the supplement's powers, making it more easily accepted by the brain and body and enhancing its medicinal sleep effects.

- **Asparagus:** On top of helping to lessen mucus production and soothe inflammation, asparagus has a calming, sedative effect because it cleanses antagonizers such as free radicals and positively charged chemicals that disrupt homeostasis (balance) in the body systems. When combined with **GABA** and **magnesium L-threonate**, asparagus engages the supplements, making them more effective.

- **Spinach:** High in calcium, this is an alkaline food useful for reducing acidosis. Spinach also contains mineral salts, which feed neurotransmitters and enhance the supplement **glycine**'s absorbability—which helps strengthen neurotransmitter performance.

- **Celery:** High in mineral salts that (1) carry electrical impulses through the brain and (2) are the building blocks of neurotransmitter creation. Celery can really enhance the ability of supplemental **GABA**, **glycine**, and **magnesium L-threonate** to be absorbed by the brain and aid in neurotransmitter performance for sleep support.

- **Lettuce:** The "milk" in the core of a leaf of lettuce calms the nerves and has an overall tranquilizing, sedative effect. Coupled with **passionflower**, lettuce enhances the calming neurological effect of this herbal supplement.

- **Pomegranates:** These little jewels bind onto unwanted acids in the body, including lactic acid buildup that can result in leg and other muscle cramps during sleep. Pomegranates are also particularly anti-mucus and anti-inflammatory. When used alongside **magnesium glycinate**, pomegranates take the supplement's muscle relaxing powers to the next level.

- **Licorice root:** This herb helps support and rejuvenate the adrenals at a rapid pace. Licorice root ignites the chemical compounds of supplemental **magnesium glycinate**, which calms the adrenals so that the licorice can bring them back to vitality faster.

- **Wild blueberries:** These are great to pull out MSG and heavy metals from the brain, then drive them out of your body. The top adaptogenic, anti-mucus, anti-inflammatory, antioxidant-rich food you can eat, wild blueberries also enhance every nutrient, supplement, amino acid, you name it—so the body can make the best use of it.

- **Garlic:** A highly beneficial anti-inflammatory for mucous membranes and bronchial tubes.

Used long-term, garlic can ease breathing for undisturbed sleep. Plus, when you take **magnesium glycinate**, garlic's traces of bioavailable magnesium engage the supplement so you can experience even better breathing and more restful sleep.

- **Cilantro:** Binds onto toxic heavy metals and MSG and flushes them from your system. When you take supplemental **L-glutamine** with cilantro, it boosts MSG removal and becomes a cofactor in heavy metal detoxification.

- **Sweet potatoes:** Provide a critical form of glucose that stimulates the development of neurotransmitters such as glycine, dopamine, GABA, and serotonin, which aids in the ability to sleep. When you take supplemental **melatonin** at the same time you eat sweet potato, the sweet potato's nutrients bind onto the melatonin and help it travel to the brain more easily. Sweet potato and supplemental melatonin also have a powerful antioxidant effect that helps stop oxidation of toxic heavy metals in the brain.

THE SACRED SLEEP WINDOW

You probably won't resolve a sleep issue overnight. It will take time for your body to cleanse itself of toxins, heal, and rebuild, so in the meantime, remind yourself of the laws of sleep: that your sleep wellspring will wait for you no matter what and that you deserve to grant yourself a sleep allowance. On top of this, you can help yourself navigate whatever rocky nights come your way by holding close a secret about how sleep works. This is important to know about even if you never have trouble sleeping, because it's the key to the *best* sleep.

First, it's important to understand that you do heal even when you don't sleep. You'll hear from some sources that the body only performs true healing functions during deep sleep. Do not despair. If you are lying down with your eyes closed between the hours of 10 P.M. and 2 A.M., even if you are awake, your body is still healing. In fact, even though you are conscious, part of your brain is asleep. The part of your brain that's awake may annoy you with messages that you're falling behind from lack of sleep. You may still be tired when it's time to get up. Rest assured, though, that the portion of your brain that's sleeping is allowing for your body to reset. Let any anxiety drift out the door as you relax into the knowledge that you are still reaping some benefits of sleep.

That 10 P.M. to 2 A.M. range is a sacred window. It's the time in the night when your body does most of its healing. If you *are* able to sleep during that period, your body is healing at an accelerated rate. Even if you only catch 10 minutes, those 10 minutes will be potent. The restoration your body performs in that snippet of time will power you through on your path to healing.

As far as the ideal amount of sleep you need in a given night goes, it varies from person to person. Some can get by on five or six hours, while others do best with eight or nine. There's not one golden number that applies to everyone, though a minimum of four and a half hours will leave you in a better place than anything less. What does matter for all of us is *when* sleep occurs. If you fall asleep at 10 P.M. and wake at 5 A.M., there's a good chance you'll actually feel more rested than if you nod off at 1 A.M. and sleep for eight or nine hours. It's all about that sleep window.

Keep in mind that naps are a helpful tool and shouldn't be dismissed as childish. We all run into those days when we need a little shut-eye during daylight hours, whether because we worked a night shift, stayed up on a deadline, or simply couldn't get enough sleep the night before. For the most beneficial healing to occur, try to lie down with your eyes closed sometime between 10 A.M. and 2 P.M. That range is the daytime equivalent of the night's sacred healing window. If you use it to your advantage, you will feel all the difference.

SPIRITUAL SLEEP SUPPORT

The Angel of Sleep is always there for you if you need her. Whenever you're seeking guidance or comfort, speak her name aloud and ask for her help. She'll aid you in your path to a better night's sleep, whether because of a health issue or an emotional trial. On those nights when an unresolved issue is keeping you up, speak to the Angel of Sleep. Tell her that you're struggling with a problem that you can't process right now, because it will get in the way of your rest. She'll help put out the emotional fire so you can have some peace, and she'll help you access your sleep wellspring. More effective than any sleeping pill, the Angel of Sleep will watch over you as you travel to the land of the subconscious.

CHAPTER 31

Why Bad Dreams Are Good

Dreams are the ultimate mystery—they can't be weighed or measured. *What are dreams telling us?* we ask ourselves from the time we're children. *What do they mean?*

Especially, we question the bad dreams. What's behind the nightmares, the anger dreams, the frustration dreams, the stress dreams, the sweat dreams, the wake-in-the-night-screaming dreams? How can we make them go away? Are they punishment? Can't we have some more blissed-out dreams of tropical island vacations instead?

Once you understand what's behind those bad dreams, you won't want them to go anywhere. "Bad" dreams are the soul's way of healing. When we're awake, we're not supposed to be breaking down the walls of our emotional hurt. When we are wounded, a physical component in the brain puts up a barrier to prevent us from constantly processing and reprocessing the pain, so that we can be productive and move forward during our waking hours. They're not walls of denial; they're walls of divine protection. While some conscious processing is healthy and necessary, it's not meant to haunt us.

The time to process that pain is in our sleep. When we're not conscious, the emotional walls come down so the soul can do its cleanup and repair work. This means that all sorts of difficult emotions get stirred up, and they work themselves out through our dreams. If this didn't happen, frustration, anger, fear, betrayal, guilt, and humiliation would build up and up and up within us until they overpowered the strength of the walls holding them in place and took over our waking lives. Instead, our dreams release them. This nightly housecleaning—aided by the Angel of Sleep, the Angel of Dreams, and the Unknown Angels—helps us face what's going on in life without becoming scarred by it.

Sometimes dreams have staying power. A dream can stick to you all day or even longer—even years. These dreams can be confusing. We often dream of family and other loved ones, for example, with a swirl of emotions. Even if everything is going fine in a waking relationship, a dream can bring a feeling of hurt or uneasiness. Or if it's a relationship where's there's been some challenge or distance, dreams can bring up the old wounds, making us contemplate what went wrong years ago to cause the pain. We may wake from a dream feeling like we did something wrong, or like we weren't heard or perceived right. As we painfully try to decode what it all means, we can be left feeling empty.

All of this is healthy. I've heard from people who told me that a bad dream made them pick up the phone and call a family member or friend they hadn't talked to in years, starting a process of great healing. Any empty feeling is because toxic wounds and emotions left us (or started to leave us) in our sleep, reducing our storage bank of hurt. Even though we think it's the opposite, bad dreams rejuvenate us. They remind us that there are people, places, and things in our lives that may need some attention so we can move on. Bad dreams don't close doors; they open doors. They create new beginnings. Even if you're not aware of what that new beginning is, it's happening. Far down the road, you may have the perspective to see what opportunity a bad dream led to in your life.

We wish each other "sweet dreams," when really, we should wish each other "healing dreams." To advance the soul, mend the heart, and empty yourself of harmful emotions, you don't want every dream to be perfect and tranquil and flowery. You don't want your dream life to be an all-out wonderland. You want your dreams to have some hardship in them, because you want the good stuff to be happening when you're awake. If our dream lives were total fantasy, sleeping would be the only thing we'd want to do.

Now, there are sinister people in the world. They have existed throughout history. These coldhearted people can go through life without one nightmare. That's an indication of how cut off they are from processing negative experiences like pain and suffering. Since they don't deal with their pain while they sleep, they hold on to it in their waking lives, and they want to inflict it on others.

On the flip side, you can have the most compassionate, generous, loving person who can't go a night without dreaming something unpleasant. Believe it or not, this is the healthier process. Because this person is so tuned in, she's a witness to others' struggles. She experiences the range of human suffering, and so when she checks out for the night, her brain needs to protect her from becoming haunted by it in her waking life. She may dream of school-yard bullies and natural disasters and war zones, and it's all for her benefit—so that rather than waking up bitter that she has to leave some fantastical dream and face a harsh world instead, she can wake up relieved to leave those tough dreams behind, and ready to continue her sacred work of compassion.

Let me be clear that having good dreams does not make you a bad person. Of course not. It's all about balance. In addition to those memorable "bad" dreams, we're meant to have beautiful dreams, as well. The angels sometimes grant us dreams of transcendence and hope. Sometimes our dreams are premonitions or messages or creative inspiration. Some nights, we have mild bad dreams in which we process emotions, though we're spared from remembering what happened come morning. Other times, we get to visit with a deceased loved one in our dreams.

Just remember to welcome, too, the dreams that challenge you—they are doing you a great service as your body heals during slumber. They are not a punishment or judgment. They are helping you become your best self.

Afterword
Your Soul's Gold

Since gold was discovered, it has had a magnetic pull on us, one that goes far beyond any monetary worth.

As a child, did you ever wish for a gold star on your paper at school? It wasn't because you could take it to the pawn shop and get cash for it. You yearned for that cheap sticker because of what it represented: achievement, worthiness, approval.

If you have a grandmother's favorite locket or ring, again, it's not the dollar figure behind that gold that gives it a special place in your heart. It's the spiritual meaning: appreciation, nostalgia, loyalty, love.

And do Olympians go for the gold because of the market value of the metal? No, they spend their whole lives training to win because of what the prize stands for: blood, sweat, tears, spirit, will, intention, and sacrifice that come together into a moment of human greatness.

When spiritual and emotional meaning are connected to a piece of gold or other treasure, its worth is on a level above price tags. The Knights Templar went searching for the Holy Grail not because of the money they'd get for this gold vessel but because of the mystical significance it was said to hold as the cup Jesus drank from at the Last Supper. Though the knights turned up hundreds upon hundreds of gold cups, they were cast off as worthless because they didn't hold the power. It was all about the spiritual meaning.

I'm here to tell you that you don't have to go on an epic quest, earn anyone's approval, inherit a family heirloom, learn to high-jump, or have an overflowing bank account in order to claim the world's most precious treasure. Gold, platinum, diamonds, sapphires, the Holy Grail, the Ark of the Covenant, Noah's ark, even the Beatles' lost album—none of these hold a candle to your soul's gold and gems and jewels that you already carry inside of you.

Yes, you. I know it's been a struggle to deal with health problems or great loss or hardship. I understand what you might have suffered as you wondered if you were aging before your time, if your thyroid was calling it quits, and if your body was giving up on you—or even working against you. I can only imagine what you've gone through in your search for answers.

It's probably left you defeated at times, lonely, despairing, and doubtful of your own worth. Know this: It's not your fault; you didn't deserve any of it. You didn't create your illness or imagine it. You're not a bad person. You *can* heal and move forward.

All that time that symptoms were limiting you, they were giving you something, too. That compassion you gained from being vulnerable, that wisdom that came from watching life at a distance, that faith that there had to be an answer, that supreme patience of putting one foot in front of the other—these are yours to use for the rest of your life. Losses, struggles, wounds, suffering, pain, sorrow, fear, hardships, trials, letdowns, and battles are not what any of us would choose. When they visit us, though, we get our greatest tools and treasures.

Those tools and treasures can be heavy. To be in touch with the world's suffering is not easy. Just like a bag of diamonds and gold, it can weigh you down. Which is why it's time for you to come into the spiritual significance of your challenges—because when you attach spiritual meaning to your treasures, it makes them light as light itself.

You've been picked out of the crowd as a special person who can change the world. Because you hold power, illness tried to hold you back. You probably experienced symptoms along the way, and this may have gotten you labeled with a whole bunch of different names for what was supposedly wrong with you. Yet the plan of you being picked on backfired. Instead of being constrained, you were pushed forward and forced to grow and develop in your soul and spirit. You gained understandings and insights that brought you closer to God.

Now you get to rid yourself of your illness and all those symptoms and labels that have come with it. You get to heal, rise above, and reclaim your power—power that's more than you know.

Your thyroid, that part of your body you may have once been led to believe was your weakest point or even your enemy, has in fact been your greatest strength and protector. This gland doesn't operate only on a physical level. Spiritually, it's your shield, your guard watching over all those treasures you've earned—part of your armor as you go through life. The armored guards protecting the gold at Fort Knox have nothing on your thyroid.

Through everything that has happened to it, even through surgery or radioactive iodine treatment, your thyroid's spirit has remained. It's been there all along, looking out for you. It's held on to those treasures, waiting for the day you'd discover them. As you bring your thyroid and the rest of your body back to health, you'll be supporting it even more in taking care of your soul's wealth—wealth you will use to spread divine light to everyone around you.

No matter who you are or where you come from, what you've done or think you have not done, know that through the true living words in this book, Spirit and I will always be there for you.

Remember: You are a world changer. Spirit and I see and hear you. We believe in you. We stand beside you. And we can't wait for you to experience what's next.

ENDNOTES

1. M. A. Epstein, M. D. Cantab, B. G. Achong, and Y. M. Barr, "Virus Particles in Cultured Lymphoblasts from Burkitt's Lymphoma," *The Lancet* 283, no. 7335 (1964): 702–703, doi: 10.1016/S0140-6736(64)91524-7

2. "History of the Great Lakes Water Quality Agreement," Environmental and Climate Change Canada, accessed Dec 18, 2016, https://www.canada.ca/en/environment-climate-change/services/great-lakes-protection/canada-united-states-water-quality-agreement/overview.html; "Lake Erie," United States Environmental Protection Agency (EPA), last updated May 4, 2016, https://www.epa.gov/greatlakes/lake-erie.

INDEX

Note: Page numbers in italics indicate recipes. Page numbers in parentheses indicate noncontiguous references.

M

Magnesium, 151. *See also* Asparagus; Celery; Mangoes
Magnesium glycinate, 256
Magnesium, lack of, 51, 52, 251
Manganese, 152. *See also* Nuts
Mangoes, 144, *192, 200, 225,* 255
Maple syrup, 144, *188, 222*
Mason Jar Salads Two Ways, *198*
Medications
    overprescribed, as virus triggers, 12
    thyroid. *See* Thyroid medication
    "virus-friendly" prescriptions as virus triggers, 12
Melatonin, 255. *See also* Sweet potatoes
Memory loss, 27, 47, 57, 85
Ménière's disease, 53–54
Menopause. *See* Perimenopause and menopause
Menstrual periods, abnormal, 39, 55–56, 57, 59
Mercury. *See also* Toxic heavy metals
    ADHD and, 27
    antidotes for removing, 142, 149, 150
    brain fog and, 47
    connective tissue disorders and, 53
    dental amalgams, 10, 11
    excessive sweating and, 48
    forms of, 11
    hysteria from, 120
    inherited from parents, 114
    irritability and, 50
    memory loss and, 47
    metallic taste in mouth and, 54
    as thyroid virus trigger, 11, 19
    trembling hands and, 52
    twitches, spasms and, 52
Metabolism
    cold sensitivity (heightened) and, 47
    mystery weight gain and, 42, 109–110
    myth of, as Great Mistake, 109–111
    problems, 41–42
    thyroid hormones and, 32
    thyroid's purpose and, 31
Metallic taste in mouth, 54
Migraines, 27, 51, 67, 122
Miscarriage, 57–59
Mold, 11, 14, 36
Monolaurin, 150
Mononucleosis and mono symptoms, 18, 20, 21–22, 23–24, 37, 58–59, 94,

143, 149–150
Mood swings, 49, 66
MSG toxicity, 248
MTHF. *See* 5-MTHF
MTHFR gene mutation, 60, 148
    Multiple sclerosis (MS), 62
Muscle cramps, 51, 256
Muscle weakness, 51
Mushrooms, *214*
Mushrooms, Chaga, 150
Myalgic encephalomyelitis (ME), 61
Mystery illness
    first instances of symptoms, 36–37
    misconception, Great Mistake of, 101
    stage of EBV, 26–29

N

"Nachos-Style" Baked Potatoes, *208*
Nails, brittle/ridged, 54–55
Nettle leaf, 150–151
Neurotoxins, viral
    aches, pains and, 51
    anxiety and, 50, 251
    blurry/other vision problems and, 56
    brain fog and, 47
    celiac disease and, 64
    characteristics of, 19–20
    chest tightness and, 53
    chronic fatigue syndrome, related maladies and, 61
    cold hands/feet and, 48
    cold sensitivity (heightened) and, 47, 99
    connective tissue disorders and, 63
    constipation and, 55
    decreasing production of, healing and, 158
    energy level changes and, 47
    excessive sweating and, 48
    eye floaters and, 56
    fatigue and, 46, 99
    fibromyalgia and, 61
    foods for protecting from, 141–142, 143, 144, 145, 147
    gluten mystery misery and, 136
    headaches, migraines and, 51
    heartbeat irregularities and, 52–53
    insomnia and, 241–242, 251
    irritability and, 50
    lupus and, 62
    metallic taste in mouth and, 54
    mood swings and, 49
    multiple sclerosis (MS) and, 62
    muscle weakness and, 51

mystery illness stage and, 27
mystery weight gain and, 42
non-healing injuries and, 61
plantar fasciitis and, 65
potency of, 20
Raynaud's syndrome and, 65
restless legs and, 50–51
restlessness and, 50
sense of taste/smell altered and, 54
sleep apnea and, 254
supplements for protecting from, 148, 149, 150, 152
swollen hands/feet and, 49
throat tightness and, 54
thyroid cancer and, 71
thyroid stage of EBV and, 24
tingles, numbness and, 51–52
tinnitus and, 53
trembling hands and, 52
twitches, spasms and, 52
vertigo, Ménière's disease, dizziness, balance issues and, 53–54
90-Day Thyroid Rehab, 153–161
    about: overview and selection of Choices, 153–155
    Choice A: Liver, Lymphatic, and Gut Release Month, 155–156
    Choice B: Heavy Metal Detox Month, 157–158
    Choice C: Thyroid Virus Cleanse Month, 159–161
Nodules, cysts, and tumors. *See also* Thyroid cancer
    autoimmune link, 29
    description and meaning of symptoms, 41
    EBV and, 18, 23, 26, 41
    foods/supplements to help, (140–142), (144–150), 225, 226
    healed, one woman's story, 231–233
    parathyroid disease and, 66
    removal of thyroid and, 129–130
Noodles, pesto zucchini, *196*
Numbness and tingles, 51–52, 142. *See also* Raynaud's syndrome
Nuts, 144–145, 160, *184, 196, 198,* (*208–212*), *214, 220. See also* Almond flour

O

Onions and scallions, 145, *180, 198, 208, 210, 214, 218*
Oranges and tangerines, 145, *190, 192, 200, 202, 226*

Z

ACKNOWLEDGMENTS

Thank you to Patty Gift, Anne Barthel, Reid Tracy, Margarete Nielsen, Diane Hill, everyone at Hay House Radio, and the rest of the Hay House team for your faith and commitment to getting Spirit of Compassion's wisdom out into the world so it can continue to change lives.

Hilary Swank and Philip Schneider, your dedication to the healing truth and wisdom is remarkable, and I am deeply honored. Your support is immensely powerful.

Helen Lasichanh and Pharrell Williams, you are extraordinarily kindhearted seers.

Sylvester Stallone, Jennifer Flavin Stallone, and family, your support has been legendarily game-changing.

Kate Hudson, Danny Fujikawa, Erinn and Oliver Hudson, and Elisabeth Stassen, having you guys on my side with your love and support is a blessing.

Miranda Kerr and Evan Spiegel, it's so amazing to have your hands of light and compassion behind the healing movement.

Laura Dern, thank you for spreading your light and changing the world for the better.

Novak and Jelena Djokovic, you are pioneers in advancing health and teaching the world how to thrive.

Gwyneth Paltrow, Elise Loehnen, and your devoted GOOP crew, your caring and generosity are a profound inspiration.

Uma Thurman, I deeply value and treasure our friendship.

Robert Downey, Jr., you're truly all heart and soul.

Sage and Tony Robbins, it's an honor to be part of your world that's helping so many.

Martin, Jean, Elizabeth, and Jacqueline Shafiroff, thank you for always being there, believing in me, and helping to spread the message so that others can heal.

Dr. Alejandro Junger, life would not be the same without you, brother.

Dr. Ilana Zablozki-Amir, your willingness to support the Medical Medium cause is epic.

Dr. Christiane Northrup, your inexhaustible devotion to the health of womankind has become its own star in the universe.

Dr. Prudence Hall, your selfless work to enlighten patients who need answers renews the true, heroic meaning of the word doctor.

Craig Kallman, thank you for your support, advocacy, and friendship on this journey.

Caroline Fleming, you're truly a blessing because you have the gift to always care about everyone around you as you share your light.

Chelsea Field and Scott, Wil, and Owen Bakula, how did I get so blessed to have you in my life? You are true crusaders for the Medical Medium cause.

Kimberly and James Van Der Beek, there's a special place in my heart for you and your family. I'm truly thankful to have crossed paths with you in this lifetime.

Kerri Walsh Jennings, you truly amaze me with your hopeful nature and endless positive energy.

John Donovan, it's an honor to be on the planet with such a peace-seeking soul.

Nanci Chambers and David James, Stephanie, and Wyatt Elliott, I can't thank you enough for your dear friendship and everlasting encouragement.

Suze Orman and KT, your determination and commitment are exceptional.

Lisa Gregorisch-Dempsey, your acts of kindness have been deeply meaningful.

Grace Hightower De Niro, Robert De Niro, and family, you are precious, gracious beings.

Liv Tyler, it's such a great honor to be a part of your world.

Jenna Dewan, your fighting spirit is an inspiration to behold.

Debra Messing, you are bettering people's lives with your vision for a healthy planet.

Alexis Bledel, your strength in this world is extraordinarily heartening.

Lisa Rinna, thank you for tirelessly using your influence to spread the message.

Jennifer Aniston, your kindness, caring, and support are on another level.

Taylor Schilling, what a joy to know you and have your support.

Marcela Valladolid, knowing you is a gift in my life.

Kelly Noonan and Alec Gores, thank you for always looking out for me. It means so much.

Jennifer Meyer, I'm beyond grateful for your friendship and how you're always spreading the word.

Calvin Harris, you've changed the world with a powerful rhythm.

Courteney Cox, thank you for having such a pure, loving heart.

Hunter Mahan and Kandi Harris, I'm proud of you for always being game to take on a challenge.

Kidada Jones and Rashida Jones, the deep care and compassion you bring to life mean more than you know. Your mother was a treasure who lives on in you.

Andrew Kusatsu: love you, brother, for persevering past the pain and fighting for health freedom.

To the following special souls whose loyalty I treasure, my thanks go out: Naomi Campbell; Eva Longoria; Lewis Howes; Carla Gugino; Mario Lopez; Renee Bargh; Tanika Ray; Maria Menounos; Michael Bernard Beckwith; Jay Shetty; Alex Kushneir; LeAnn Rimes Cibrian; Hana Hollinger; Sharon Levin; Nena, Robert, and Uma Thurman; Jenny Mollen; Jessica Seinfeld; Kelly Osbourne; Demi Moore; Kyle Richards; India.Arie; Kristen Bower; Rozonda Thomas; Peggy Rometo; Debbie Gibson; Carol, Scott, and Christiana Ritchie; Jamie-Lynn Sigler; Amanda de Cadenet; Marianne Williamson; Erin Johnson; Gabrielle Bernstein; Sophia Bush; Maha Dakhil; Bhavani Lev and Bharat Mitra; Woody Fraser, Milena Monrroy, Midge Hussey, and everyone at Hallmark's Home & Family; Morgan Fairchild; Patti Stanger; Catherine, Sophia, and Laura Bach; Annabeth Gish; Robert Wisdom; Danielle LaPorte; Nick and Brenna Ortner; Jessica

Ortner; Mike Dooley; Kris Carr; Kate Northrup; Ann Louise Gittleman; Jan and Panache Desai; Ami Beach and Mark Shadle; Brian Wilson; John Holland; Jill Black Zalben; Alexandra Cohen; Christine Hill; Carol Donahue; Caroline Leavitt; Michael Sandler and Jessica Lee; Koya Webb; Jenny Hutt; Adam Cushman; Sonia Choquette; Colette Baron-Reid; Denise Linn; and Carmel Joy Baird. I deeply value you all.

To the compassionate doctors and other healers of the world who have changed the lives of so many: I have tremendous respect for you. Dr. Masha Kogan, Dr. Virginia Romano, Dr. Habib Sadeghi, Dr. Carol Lee, Dr. Richard Sollazzo, Dr. Jeff Feinman, Dr. Deanna Minich, Dr. Ron Steriti, Dr. Nicole Galante, Dr. Diana Lopusny, Dr. Dick and Noel Shepard, Dr. Aleksandra Phillips, Dr. Chris Maloney, Drs. Tosca and Gregory Haag, Dr. Dave Klein, Dr. Deborah Kern, Dr. Darren and Suzanne Boles, and Dr. Robin Karlin—it's an honor to call you friends. Thank you for your endless dedication to the field of healing.

Thanks to David Schmerler, Kimberly S. Grimsley, and Susan G. Etheridge for being there for me.

A very warm, heartfelt thanks to Muneeza Ahmed; Kimberly Spair; Amber Stone; Lauren Henry; Kayla Botelho; Tara Tom; Bella; Victoria and Michael Arnstein; Nina Leatherer; Michelle Sutton; Haily Cataldo; Kerry; Amy Bacheller; Michael McMenamin; Alexandra Laws; Ester Horn; Linda and Robert Coykendall; Setareh Khatibi; Heather Coleman; Glenn Klausner; Michael Monteleone; Bobbi and Leslie Hall; Katherine Belzowski; Matt and Vanessa Houston; David, Holly, and Ginnie Whitney; Melody Lee Pence; Terra Appelman; Eileen Crispell; Kristin Cassidy; Calvin Stebbins; Catherine Lawton; Alana DiNardo; Min Lee; and Eden Epstein Hill.

Thank you to the countless people, including those in the Medical Medium communities, whom I've had the privilege and honor of seeing blossom, heal, and transform.

Sally Arnold, thank you for shining your light so brightly and lending your voice to the movement.

Ruby Scattergood, your masterful patience and countless hours of dedication have heroically formed the true spine of this book. The Medical Medium series would not be possible without your writing and editing. Thank you for your literary counsel.

Vibodha and Tila Clark, your creative genius has been astoundingly instrumental to the cause of helping others. Thank you for standing with us throughout the years.

Friar and Clare: *Behold, he cometh with clouds; and every eye shall see him, and they also which pierced him: and all kindreds of the earth shall wail because of him. Even so, Amen* (Rev. 1:7).

Quincy: Thank you for your invaluable support and hard work.

Sepideh Kashanian and Ben, thank you for your warm, loving care.

Oliver Niño and Mandy Morris, so proud of you for all you do for so many.

Jeff Skeirik, thank you for the best pictures, man.

Alyssa Degati, you are changing lives with your voice.

Jon Morelli and Noah, you two are all heart.

Robby Barbaro, your unwavering positivity lifts up everyone around you.

For your love and support, as always, I thank my family: my luminous wife; Dad and Mom; my brothers, nieces, nephews, aunts, and uncles; my champions Indigo, Ruby, and Great

Blue; Hope; Marjorie and Robert; Laura; Rhia and Byron; Alayne Serie and Scott, Perri, Lissy, and Ari Cohn; David Somoroff; Joel, Liz, Kody, Jesse, Lauren, Joseph, and Thomas; Brian, Joyce, and Josh; Jarod; Brent; Kelly and Evy; Danielle, Johnny, and Declan; and all my loved ones who are on the other side.

Finally, thank you, Spirit of the Most High (aka Spirit of Compassion), for providing all of us with compassionate wisdom from the heavens that inspires us to keep our heads up and carry the sacred gifts you've been so kind to give us. Thank you for putting up with me over the years and reminding me to keep a light heart with your never-ending patience and willingness to answer my questions in search of the truth.

ABOUT THE AUTHOR

Anthony William is the originator of the global celery juice movement, host of the *Medical Medium Podcast*, and #1 *New York Times* best-selling author of the Medical Medium book series:

- *Medical Medium Cleanse to Heal: Healing Plans for Sufferers of Anxiety, Depression, Acne, Eczema, Lyme, Gut Problems, Brain Fog, Weight Issues, Migraines, Bloating, Vertigo, Psoriasis, Cysts, Fatigue, PCOS, Fibroids, UTI, Endometriosis & Autoimmune*

- *Medical Medium Celery Juice: The Most Powerful Medicine of Our Time Healing Millions Worldwide*

- *Medical Medium Liver Rescue: Answers to Eczema, Psoriasis, Diabetes, Strep, Acne, Gout, Bloating, Gallstones, Adrenal Stress, Fatigue, Fatty Liver, Weight Issues, SIBO & Autoimmune Disease*

- *Medical Medium Thyroid Healing: The Truth behind Hashimoto's, Graves', Insomnia, Hypothyroidism, Thyroid Nodules & Epstein-Barr*

- *Medical Medium Life-Changing Foods: Save Yourself and the Ones You Love with the Hidden Healing Powers of Fruits & Vegetables*

- *Medical Medium: Secrets Behind Chronic and Mystery Illness and How to Finally Heal*

Anthony was born with the unique ability to converse with the Spirit of Compassion, who provides him with extraordinarily advanced healing medical information that's far ahead of its time. Since age four, Anthony has been using his gift to see into people's conditions and tell them and their doctors how to recover their health. His unprecedented accuracy and success rate as the Medical Medium have earned him the trust and love of millions worldwide, among them movie stars, rock stars, billionaires, professional athletes, and countless other people from all walks of life who couldn't find a way to heal until he provided them with insights from above. Over the decades, Anthony has also been an invaluable resource to doctors who need help solving their most difficult cases.

Learn more at www.medicalmedium.com.

Hay House Titles of Related Interest

YOU CAN HEAL YOUR LIFE, the movie,
starring Louise Hay & Friends
(available as an online streaming video)
www.hayhouse.com/louise-movie

THE SHIFT, the movie,
starring Dr. Wayne W. Dyer
(available as an online streaming video)
www.hayhouse.com/the-shift-movie

———

*MEDICAL MEDIUM: Secrets behind Chronic and Mystery Illness
and How to Finally Heal,* by Anthony William

*MEDICAL MEDIUM LIFE-CHANGING FOODS: Save Yourself and the Ones You Love
with the Hidden Healing Powers of Fruits & Vegetables,* by Anthony William

*MEDICAL MEDIUM LIVER RESCUE: Answers to Eczema, Psoriasis, Diabetes, Strep,
Acne, Gout, Bloating, Gallstones, Adrenal Stress, Fatigue, Fatty Liver, Weight Issues,
SIBO & Autoimmune Disease,* by Anthony William

*MEDICAL MEDIUM CELERY JUICE: The Most Powerful Medicine of
Our Time Healing Millions Worldwide,* by Anthony William

*MEDICAL MEDIUM CLEANSE TO HEAL: Healing Plans for Sufferers of Anxiety,
Depression, Acne, Eczema, Lyme, Gut Problems, Brain Fog, Weight Issues,
Migraines, Bloating, Vertigo, Psoriasis, Cysts, Fatigue, PCOS, Fibroids, UTI,
Endometriosis & Autoimmune,* by Anthony William

All of the above are available at your local bookstore,
or may be ordered by contacting Hay House (see next page).

———